Aches To Assets

Orange Books Publication

1st Floor, Rajhans Arcade, Mall Road, Kohka, Bhilai, Chhattisgarh 490020
Website: **www.orangebooks.in**

© **Copyright, 2025, Author**

All rights reserved. No part of this book may be reproduced, stored in a retrieval system, or transmitted, in any form by any means, electronic, mechanical, magnetic, optical, chemical, manual, photocopying, recording or otherwise, without the prior written consent of its writer.

First Edition, 2025

ISBN: 978-93-6554-949-2

ACHES TO ASSETS

HOW PAIN BECAME A BILLION DOLLAR SCAM

DR. SAHITYA GOTETY

**INTERVENTIONAL PAIN SPECIALIST,
M.B.B.S. DNB, FIAPM, FIPM**

Orange Books Publication
www.orangebooks.in

Introduction

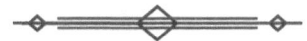

Aches To Assets: Turning Pain Into Possibility

Pain. A word that carries more weight than it seems. It doesn't just affect your body—it infiltrates your emotions, your relationships, and even your sense of purpose. As a pain specialist, I've seen how this silent invader forces people to give up what they cherish—whether it's playing with their children, pursuing their passions, or simply living a day without discomfort.

But pain isn't just a personal battle. It's also a business. Hospitals run like corporations, treatments are influenced by profit-driven strategies, and doctors often find themselves caught between genuine care and the pressure to meet commercial expectations. This book, "Aches to Assets," takes a deeper look at how pain—both personal and systemic—can be transformed into something meaningful.

Here, "assets" carry multiple meanings. On a personal level, it's about reclaiming your life and turning struggles into strength. From a business perspective, it's a candid exploration of how pain is often monetized, how healthcare is becoming commercialized, and what that means for patients and doctors alike.

I didn't always plan to specialize in pain. Like many medical students, I envisioned a career in surgery or cardiology. But during my rotations, I noticed one thing—pain was everywhere, yet rarely addressed with the seriousness it deserved. It wasn't just a symptom; for many, it was the problem. That realization drove me to focus on pain management, not just as a doctor but as someone who could advocate for better care and ethical practices in the medical industry.

This book is for anyone who has felt trapped by pain—whether physical, emotional, or systemic. You'll learn about cutting-edge treatments, practical strategies for managing pain, and how to navigate the complexities of modern healthcare. But more than that, it's about pulling back the curtain on how the medical industry works.

Pain is complex, but it doesn't have to define your life. Whether you're someone seeking relief or a professional striving to make a difference in this field, this book will help you see how pain can be turned into progress—not just for individuals but for the system as a whole.

Let's embark on this journey together, turning aches into assets and finding hope that lies on the other side.

With hope and healing,

*~ **Dr. Sahitya***

Contents

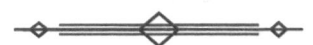

Part 1
Understanding Pain

Chapter 1
The Anatomy Of Pain 2
1.1 The Science Behind Pain 2
1.2 How The Brain Processes Pain 5
1.3 Pain Signals: Acute Vs. Chronic 9
1.4 Hidden Triggers Of Pain 14
1.5 The Psychological Dimensions Of Pain 20

Chapter 2
Pain And Its Causes 27
2.1 Common Chronic Pain Conditions 27
2.2 Lifestyle And Environmental Factors 33
2.3 How Poor Posture Causes Pain 39
2.4 Hormonal Impact Of Pain In Women 43
2.5 Pain In The Elderly: Unique Challenges 47

Chapter 3

Innovations In Pain Relief 54

3.1 Cutting-Edge Technology In
Pain Management 54

3.2 Stem Cells And Regenerative Medicine 59

3.3 The Future Of Non-Surgical Techniques 63

3.4 Artificial Intelligence In Diagnostics 66

3.5 Robotics-Assisted Pain Relief 67

Part 2
The Physician's Perspective

Chapter 4

Life As A Pain Specialist 71

4.1 A Day In The Life Of A Pain Physician 71

4.2 Challenges In Treating Chronic
Pain Patients... 73

4.3 The Emotional Toll Of Dealing
With Suffering 77

4.4 Building Trust With Patients 81

4.5 Balancing Professional
And Personal Life 84

Chapter 5

Social Media And Medicine 87

5.1 The Double-Edged Sword Of
Social Media In Healthcare................................. 87

5.2 Misinformation About Pain And Its Impact 88

   5.3 The Rise Of Internet Doctors
       And Their Influence.. 89

   5.4 Building A Credible Online
       Presence As A Doctor.. 90

   5.5 How Social Media Shapes
       Patient Expectations... 92

Chapter 6
The Medical Industry Ecosystem 94

   6.1 Medical Representatives :
       Incentives And Ethics.. 94

   6.2 Navigating The Grey Areas
       Of Medical Marketing 99

   6.3 Balancing Evidence-Based
       Medicine And Patient Demands 101

   6.4 Surgeons Vs. Pain Physicians:
       Collaborations Et Conflicts 104

Part 3
Empowering Patients

Chapter 7
Taking Charge Of Your Pain 110

   7.1 Patient Education: Understanding
       Your Condition 110

   7.2 How To Communicate Effectively
       With Your Doctor... 112

   7.3 Setting Realistic Goals For Pain Relief........... 116

   7.4 Pain Diaries: A Tool For Tracking
       And Managing Pain 121

   7.5 Red Flags That Need Urgent
       Medical Attention 126

Chapter 8

Myths And Facts About Pain 132

   8.1 Debunking Common Myths
       About Pain Relief 132

   8.2 Understanding The Role Of
       Injections In Pain Management 137

   8.3 Can Yoga or Home Remedies
       Replace Medical Treatment? 144

   8.4 The Truth About Supplements
       And Alternative Medicine 147

Part 4

A Holistic Approach To Pain Relief

Chapter 9

The Role Of Mind-Body Connection 154

   9.1 How Stress Amplifies Pain 154

   9.2 Rewiring The Brain For Pain Tolerance 160

Chapter 10

Lifestyle As Medicine 167

   10.1 Nutrition's Role In Pain Management 167

   10.2 Ergonomics: How To Create
        A Pain-Free Workspace 172

10.3 The Role Of Physical Activity 178
  10.4 Quality Sleep And Its
       Impact On Pain Relief 184
  10.5 Preventing Pain Through
       Daily Habits 187

Part 5
Behind The Scenes In Medicine

Chapter 11
The Art Of Diagnosis 193
  11.1 Listening To The Patient's Story 193
  11.2 Identifying Patterns And
       Rare Conditions 198

Chapter 12
The Business Of Healthcare 204
  12.1 Challenges Of Running
       A Pain Clinic 204
  12.2 The Economics Of Non-
       Surgical Treatments 208
  12.3 The Impact Of Corporate
       Hospitals On Specialists 213
  12.4 Is Healthcare Becoming
       Too Commercial? 218

Part 6
Inspiration And Legacy

Chapter 13
Breaking The Pain Cycle 224

13.1 The Importance Of
Early Intervention 224

13.2 Building A Support System
For Chronic Pain Patients 226

13.3 Overcoming Stigma Around
Pain And Treatment 227

13.4 For All The Aspiring Doctors 228

Part 1
Understanding Pain

Chapter 1
The Anatomy Of Pain

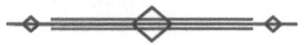

1.1 The Science Behind Pain

Pain is universal, universal yet deeply personal. It's something we all experience at some point in our lives—be it the sting of a paper cut, the ache of a sore muscle, or the relentless throb of a migraine. But have you ever stopped to wonder what pain truly is? What's happening inside your body when you feel it?

At its core, pain is your body's way of saying, *"Pay attention! Something's wrong."* It's a protective mechanism designed to alert you to injury, illness, or danger. While it can be unpleasant (and often unbearable), pain is an essential survival tool. Without it, we wouldn't know to pull our hand away from a hot stove or to stop walking with a sprained ankle.

Let's take a closer look at the fascinating science behind pain.

What Is Pain? A Protective Mechanism

Pain isn't just a feeling; it's a complex interaction between your nervous system, brain, and body. Think of it as your body's alarm system. When you stub your toe or scrape your knee, specialized nerve endings called

nociceptors are activated. These nociceptors detect damage to your tissues and send electrical signals through your nerves to your spinal cord. From there, the signals are relayed to your brain, which interprets them as pain.

This entire process happens in milliseconds. It's your body's way of ensuring you react quickly to potential harm. But here's where it gets interesting: not all pain is created equal. The intensity, duration, and even experience of pain can vary widely, depending on the type of injury, your emotional state, and even your past experiences.

The Nervous System's Role

Your nervous system is like a highway, with nerves acting as the roads that carry information between your body and brain. Pain signals travel along two main types of nerves:

- **A-Delta Fibers:** These are the speed demons of the nervous system. They carry sharp and immediate pain signals—such as the sting of a needle or the burn of hot water.

- **C Fibers:** Slower and steadier, these nerves are responsible for dull, aching pain, such as the soreness you feel after a workout.

Once the signals reach your spinal cord, they're sent to the brain for interpretation. But here's the kicker: your brain doesn't just *receive* pain signals; it can also *amplify* or *dampen* them.

The Brain's Role In Pain Perception

Pain isn't just physical—it's a sensory and emotional experience. That's why two people can have a completely different reaction to the same injury. For example, a professional athlete might brush off a sprained ankle and keep playing, while someone else might feel immobilized by the same injury.

This variability is due to how the brain processes pain. Several key areas of the brain are involved:

- **Thalamus**: Acts as the relay station, directing pain signals to the appropriate regions.
- **Somatosensory Cortex**: Identifies where the pain is and how severe it is.
- **Limbic System**: Adds the emotional layer—why pain can make you feel frustrated, scared, or even hopeless.

Interestingly, the brain can also create pain where there is no injury at all. This phenomenon, known as **phantom pain**, occurs in people who have lost a limb but continue to feel pain in the missing body part.

Neurotransmitters And Pain

Pain doesn't just rely on nerves; it also depends on chemicals in your brain called **neurotransmitters**. These chemicals act as messengers, helping pain signals travel between nerves. Some neurotransmitters, like glutamate and substance P, amplify pain signals, while others, like serotonin and endorphins, help reduce them.

This is why activities like exercise, meditation, and even laughter can sometimes reduce pain—they increase the production of natural painkillers like endorphins.

Why Understanding Pain Matters

By understanding the science behind pain, we can better manage it. Whether it's acute pain from an injury or chronic pain from conditions like arthritis, knowing how pain works is the first step toward finding relief.

In the chapters ahead, we'll explore how pain evolves, why it becomes chronic for some people and the strategies we can use to break free from its grip. For now, remember this: pain is a signal, not a sentence. It's your body's way of asking for attention—and with the right care, it *can* be quieted.

1.2 How The Brain Processes Pain

Pain doesn't stop at your injury—it continues its journey to your brain, where it's interpreted and understood. Think of the brain as the command center, deciding what to do with the distress signals your body sends. What's fascinating is that pain isn't just *felt*; it's processed, analyzed, and even influenced by your emotions and memories.

Let's delve into the brain's role in pain perception and why it's so much more than just a physical sensation.

The Pain Pathway: From Body To Brain

When you touch something sharp or sprain an ankle, pain signals begin their journey at the site of injury. Here's how they travel:

1. **Nociceptors Detect Damage:** These specialized nerve endings sense injury and generate electrical signals.
2. **The Spinal Cord Acts As A Relay Station:** Pain signals travel through peripheral nerves to the spinal cord, where they are analyzed and either amplified or suppressed.
3. **The Brain Takes Over:** The signals then move to the brain, where they are processed and interpreted.

Pain signals travel quickly through this pathway, known as the synaptic tract, to reach the brain.

Regions Of The Brain Involved In Pain

Pain doesn't register in just one part of the brain—it's a multi-regional process involving several key areas:

- **Thalamus**: Think of it as the brain's traffic controller. The thalamus receives pain signals from the spinal cord and directs them to the appropriate regions.
- **Somatosensory Cortex**: This is where the brain pinpoints *where* the pain is and determines its intensity.
- **Limbic System**: Pain isn't just physical; it's emotional too. The limbic system adds an emotional layer, which is why chronic pain can lead to feelings of despair or anger.
- **Prefrontal Cortex**: This region is involved in decision-making and can influence how we react

to pain—whether we choose to endure it, ignore it, or seek help.

Why Pain Feels Different For Everyone

Pain is subjective, meaning no two people experience it in the same way. This variability comes down to how each person's brain processes and interprets pain signals.

- **Past Experiences**: If you've endured a similar injury before, your brain might anticipate the pain, intensifying your perception.
- **Emotions And Stress**: Anxiety, fear, or depression can amplify pain by increasing activity in the limbic system. Conversely, a calm and relaxed state can reduce pain intensity.
- **Genetics**: Some people are genetically predisposed to feel pain more acutely due to differences in their nervous systems.

The Role Of The Brain In Chronic Pain

Chronic pain isn't just a lingering version of acute pain—it's a condition in itself. Over time, the brain can become overly sensitive to pain signals, a phenomenon known as **central sensitization**. Here's how it happens:

- **The Brain Learns Pain**: Repeated exposure to pain can cause the brain to "memorize" it, even after the injury has healed.
- **Neuroplasticity In Pain**: The brain's ability to rewire itself means it can create new pathways that make pain feel more intense and harder to ignore.

- **Phantom Pain**: In cases like amputations, the brain can generate pain signals even in the absence of an injury.

Chronic pain is complex, but understanding its neurological roots can pave the way for effective treatments.

When The Brain Is The Culprit

Not all pain originates in the body—sometimes, the brain itself is the source.

- **Psychogenic Pain**: This type of pain has no clear physical cause but is very real to the person experiencing it. Stress, trauma, or mental health issues often play a role.

- **Somatization**: When emotional distress manifests as physical pain, such as headaches or stomach - aches.

The brain's ability to create pain highlights the powerful connection between mind and body.

Managing Pain Through The Brain

The brain isn't just a passive recipient of pain signals—it can also help manage and reduce them. Techniques like **mindfulness meditation, cognitive-behavioural therapy (CBT),** and even simple practices like deep breathing can "rewire" the brain to handle pain more effectively.

Research shows that practices like meditation can reduce activity in the brain's pain-processing regions, making it a powerful tool for managing chronic pain.

Pain: A Brain-Body Dialogue

Pain is far more than a physical sensation—it's a dialogue between your body and brain. Understanding this relationship is crucial for both patients and healthcare providers. When we address not just the source of pain but also how the brain processes it, we open up new possibilities for relief and healing.

This is the foundation of pain management: acknowledging the brain's central role and working with it, not against it.

1.3 Pain Signals: Acute Vs. Chronic

Pain might seem like a straightforward sensation, but it's incredibly nuanced. At its most basic level, pain can be categorized into two main types: **acute** and **chronic**. While both types share the same goal—to alert the body to a problem—they differ significantly in how they manifest, how long they last, and how they affect the person experiencing them.

In this chapter, let's explore the difference between acute and chronic pain, why some pain becomes persistent, and the implications this has for treatment.

What Is Acute Pain?

Acute pain is what most people think of when they hear the word *pain*. It's sudden, sharp, and often linked to an identifiable cause—like a broken bone, a burn, or surgery.

Essentially, acute pain is your body's alarm system, designed to grab your attention and make you act quickly.

Characteristics Of Acute Pain

- **Short Duration:** Acute pain usually lasts for a few seconds to a few weeks, depending on the severity of the injury or condition.

- **Clear Cause:** There's often a clear source, such as an injury, infection, or surgery.

- **Protective Function:** It serves as a warning signal, preventing further damage by encouraging rest and care.

- **Responsive To Treatment:** Acute pain generally resolves once the underlying issue is treated or healed.

Examples Of Acute Pain

- A sprained ankle during a run.
- The sharp sting of a bee sting.
- Post-surgical pain after a knee replacement.

While unpleasant, acute pain is often a temporary visitor, leaving as quickly as it arrived once the body heals.

What Is Chronic Pain?

Chronic pain, on the other hand, is like an unwelcome houseguest who refuses to leave. It persists for weeks, months, or even years—long after the initial injury or illness has healed. For some people, chronic pain becomes a lifelong condition that significantly impacts their quality of life.

Characteristics Of Chronic Pain

- **Long Duration:** Chronic pain is typically defined as pain lasting longer than three months.
- **No Clear Cause:** It often persists even after the original injury has healed, or it may arise without any apparent reason.
- **Complex Mechanisms:** It involves changes in the nervous system that make pain signals more persistent and intense.
- **Emotional Impact:** Chronic pain often leads to frustration, anxiety, and depression, creating a vicious cycle.

Examples Of Chronic Pain

- Back pain that lingers for years.
- Migraines that occur multiple times a month.
- Pain from conditions like fibromyalgia or rheumatoid arthritis.

The Transition From Acute To Chronic Pain

One of the most puzzling aspects of pain is why some acute pain evolves into chronic pain. Researchers believe this transition involves both physical and psychological factors:

1. **Nerve Sensitization:** Prolonged pain can cause the nervous system to become hyperactive, amplifying pain signals even in the absence of injury.

2. **Inflammation:** Persistent inflammation from an injury can lead to ongoing pain.
3. **Emotional Factors:** Anxiety, stress, and fear of pain can alter how the brain processes pain, making it more intense and long-lasting.
4. **Genetic Predisposition:** Some people are more genetically prone to chronic pain due to differences in their pain pathways.

This transition underscores the importance of early and effective pain management to prevent pain from becoming a chronic condition.

Why Chronic Pain Is More Than A Physical Problem

Unlike acute pain, which is mostly a physical response to injury, chronic pain often has a significant psychological component. It's not just about the body; it's about how the brain, emotions, and even societal factors interact with the experience of pain.

The Emotional Burden

- Chronic pain is exhausting, not just physically but mentally. The constant discomfort can lead to anxiety, depression, and feelings of hopelessness.
- Many people with chronic pain feel isolated, as others may struggle to understand what they're going through.

The Social and Economic Impact

- Chronic pain can affect work, relationships, and daily activities.
- The financial burden of ongoing treatments, medications, and doctor visits adds another layer of stress.

Acute Vs. Chronic Pain: A Comparison

Feature	Acute Pain	Chronic Pain
Duration	Short-term (days to weeks)	Long-term (3+ months)
Cause	Clear and identifiable	Often unclear
Function	Protective and adaptive	Maladaptive
Emotional Impact	Minimal	Significant
Treatment	Resolves with healing	Requires long-term care

Managing Acute And Chronic Pain

For Acute Pain

- **Immediate Care:** Address the injury or source of pain promptly.
- **Medications:** Over-the-counter painkillers or prescribed medications for severe pain.

- **Rest And Rehabilitation:** Allow time for the body to heal.

For Chronic Pain

- **Comprehensive Approach:** Chronic pain requires a combination of treatments, including physical therapy, medication, and psychological support.
- **Mind-Body Techniques:** Practices like mindfulness, yoga, and meditation can help manage pain and reduce stress.
- **Innovative Therapies:** Treatments like nerve blocks, regenerative medicine, or even cutting-edge interventions like neuromodulation can offer relief.

The Importance Of Differentiating Pain Types

Understanding the difference between acute and chronic pain is vital for both patients and healthcare providers. It guides the approach to treatment, ensures better outcomes, and helps patients regain control of their lives.

Acute pain is a warning. Chronic pain, however, is a call for deeper understanding and a long-term strategy.

1.4 Hidden Triggers Of Pain

Pain is often seen as a direct result of an injury or medical condition. We're conditioned to think that if we're hurting, it's because something physically wrong has occurred—like a sprained ankle, an inflamed joint, or a muscle strain. But what if I told you that pain doesn't always have an obvious cause? Some of the most persistent and baffling types of pain arise from hidden triggers—factors that may not be immediately apparent to you or your doctor.

In this chapter, we will uncover these hidden triggers, revealing how emotional, environmental, and lifestyle factors can contribute to your pain experience. Understanding these triggers is crucial for addressing pain at its root and identifying effective treatments.

1.4.1 Stress And Pain: The Vicious Cycle

Stress is one of the most common and insidious hidden triggers of pain. It's well-documented that stress can exacerbate many conditions, from headaches to back pain. But how exactly does stress lead to physical pain?

The Physiology Of Stress

When you're stressed, your body activates the **fight or flight** response, flooding your system with hormones like **adrenaline** and **cortisol**. While these hormones are essential for short-term survival, chronic stress can cause long-term tension in your muscles and joints. The more tense your body is, the more susceptible you become to pain.

Muscle Tension And Pain

When stressed, people often unconsciously tighten their muscles, particularly in areas like the neck, shoulders, and lower back. Over time, this tension leads to muscle stiffness, spasms, and pain. Conditions like **tension headaches** and **neck pain** are often aggravated by stress.

Impact On Inflammatory Response

Stress also triggers inflammation in the body, which can worsen conditions like **arthritis** or **fibromyalgia**, where inflammation plays a significant role in the pain cycle.

Psychological Impact Of Stress

Chronic stress can make you hyper-aware of your body's sensations, magnifying even minor discomforts. This hyperawareness induces anxiety, which in turn intensifies pain and complicates its management.

By addressing stress and its physical manifestations, we can break this vicious cycle, offering relief from pain that might seem to have no clear cause.

1.4.2 Sleep Deprivation And Its Impact On Pain

It's no secret that sleep is essential for physical and mental health. However, what many people don't realize is just how closely sleep deprivation is tied to pain. If you're not getting enough rest, your body's ability to heal and recover diminishes significantly, and your sensitivity to pain increases.

The Link Between Sleep and Pain Sensitivity

Studies have shown that poor sleep can lower your pain threshold, meaning you feel pain more intensely. Sleep deprivation activates the **nociceptive pathways**, making your nervous system more sensitive to pain signals. This is particularly evident in conditions like **chronic pain syndrome** and **fibromyalgia**, where disrupted sleep can make the pain feel worse.

Sleep Disorders And Pain

Conditions like **insomnia, sleep apnea,** and **restless leg syndrome** not only interfere with sleep but also contribute to heightened pain. People who suffer from these sleep disorders often experience chronic pain, which worsens as their sleep issues persist.

Restorative Sleep And Healing

On the flip side, improving your sleep hygiene can help reduce pain. Sleep is when the body repairs itself, restores tissues and rejuvenates cells. Without adequate rest, the body's natural healing processes are delayed, prolonging pain and inflammation.

1.4.3 Diet And Nutrition: The Hidden Culprits

What you eat can have a profound impact on how you feel, especially when it comes to pain. Some foods can trigger inflammation, while others can reduce it. However, many people aren't aware of how certain foods can trigger or exacerbate their pain.

Inflammatory Foods

Certain foods are known to promote inflammation in the body, which can lead to or worsen conditions like **arthritis, back pain,** and **migraine headaches**. These foods include:

- **Sugar:** Excessive sugar can lead to inflammation and insulin resistance.
- **Processed Foods:** Highly processed foods often contain unhealthy fats and chemicals that increase inflammation.

- **Refined Carbohydrates:** Foods like white bread, pasta, and baked goods are high in refined carbs, which can trigger inflammatory responses.

Anti-Inflammatory Foods

On the other hand, some foods can help reduce inflammation and alleviate pain. These include:

- **Omega-3 Fatty Acids:** Found in fatty fish like salmon, omega-3s are known to fight inflammation.
- **Fruits And Vegetables:** Rich in antioxidants, these foods can help reduce oxidative stress, which contributes to inflammation.
- **Turmeric And Ginger:** Both spices contain compounds that have natural anti-inflammatory properties.

What you eat plays a crucial role in either promoting or alleviating pain. By adjusting your diet to focus on anti-inflammatory foods, you can reduce the frequency and intensity of pain episodes.

1.4.4 Emotional And Psychological Factors

Our emotional health is often overlooked when discussing physical pain. However, there's a growing body of evidence linking emotions and pain. Psychological conditions like **anxiety**, **depression**, and **trauma** can trigger or worsen physical pain in ways that are not immediately visible.

The Role Of Anxiety And Depression

People who are anxious or depressed are more likely to experience chronic pain, and this pain can feel more intense. The emotional burden can amplify pain signals in the brain, leading to a heightened perception of discomfort.

Trauma And Pain

Past emotional trauma, especially from childhood, can manifest as physical pain later in life. Conditions like **post-traumatic stress disorder (PTSD)** are often linked to chronic pain, with symptoms manifesting as **musculoskeletal pain**, **headaches**, or **digestive issues**.

Pain And The Mind-Body Connection

The mind and body are deeply interconnected. Psychological factors can influence how the body responds to pain. By addressing emotional issues and working on mental well-being, you can make significant strides in managing physical pain.

1.4.5 Environmental And Lifestyle Factors

Finally, environmental and lifestyle factors can also be hidden contributors to pain. These are often overlooked in clinical settings but play a crucial role in both triggering and exacerbating pain.

Climate And Weather

For many people, changes in weather or climate can worsen pain. Cold weather can tighten muscles and joints, while hot and humid conditions can exacerbate conditions like **arthritis**.

Posture And Ergonomics

Poor posture, especially in people who sit for long periods or work at computers, can lead to chronic back and neck pain. Over time, bad posture can strain muscles, ligaments, and joints, leading to discomfort and pain.

Sedentary Lifestyle

Lack of physical activity is another hidden cause of pain. Sitting for extended periods or not moving enough can lead to stiffness, muscle weakness, and poor circulation, all of which contribute to pain.

Conclusion

Uncovering The Hidden Triggers

Pain is complex and multifaceted, often triggered by factors you might not immediately associate with it. Stress, sleep deprivation, poor diet, emotional health, and even your environment can all contribute to the intensity and duration of pain. By identifying and addressing these hidden triggers, we can begin to treat pain more effectively and holistically.

Understanding that pain is not just a physical sensation but a complex interplay of factors empowers you to take control of your health and find lasting relief.

1.5 The Psychological Dimensions Of Pain

Pain isn't just a physical sensation; it's an experience that affects the mind, emotions, and body. It can distort our perception of reality and influence how we interact with the world. Whether it's acute or chronic, pain has profound psychological implications that can, in turn, impact how we experience and manage physical discomfort.

In this chapter, we explore the psychological dimensions of pain, focusing on how the mind influences the perception of pain, how pain can lead to mental health issues, and how understanding these psychological aspects can enhance pain management and healing.

1.5.1 The Mind-Body Connection: How Emotions Amplify Pain

The mind and body are deeply interconnected, with emotions playing a pivotal role in how we experience pain. When we're in physical pain, it's natural to feel frustrated, anxious, or depressed. These emotions, in turn, can make the pain feel more intense. Conversely, emotional states like anxiety and depression can also heighten the perception of physical pain.

The Role Of Stress

When we experience emotional distress, our body releases stress hormones like **cortisol** and **adrenaline**, which can increase pain sensitivity. Stress activates the body's nervous system, leading to muscle tension, tightness, and inflammation, all of which can exacerbate physical pain. Chronic stress, in particular, can make pain seem more persistent and severe.

The Impact Of Depression

Depression and pain often go hand-in-hand. In fact, peoplewith chronic pain are more likely to experience depression, and vice versa. This relationship is bidirectional—pain can lead to depression, and depression can worsen pain. Depression can alter how the brain processes pain signals, making you more sensitive to discomfort.

The Role Of Anxiety

Anxiety is another psychological factor that can magnify the perception of pain. When we're anxious, our body goes into a heightened state of alertness, making us more aware of even the slightest discomfort. People with anxiety often have a lower pain threshold, meaning they feel pain more intensely.

By recognizing and addressing these emotional and psychological factors, we can better manage the physical experience of pain and break the cycle of emotional distress.

1.5.2 Pain Catastrophizing: The Power Of Negative Thoughts

One of the most influential psychological factors in pain management is the phenomenon known as **catastrophizing**. This term refers to a tendency to magnify the severity of pain and anticipate the worst possible outcomes, often without solid evidence to support those fears.

What Is Pain Catastrophizing?

Pain catastrophizing is when individuals have negative, exaggerated thoughts about their pain. They may believe the pain will never end, that they'll never be able to live a normal life again, or that the pain is a sign of something much worse. These thoughts can lead to heightened emotional distress, which in turn makes the pain feel even more unbearable.

How Catastrophizing Affects Pain

Research shows that people who engage in catastrophizing are more likely to experience long-term pain and tend to have poorer outcomes with treatment. This is because negative thought patterns increase anxiety, stress, and muscle tension, all of which make pain worse.

Breaking The Cycle Of Catastrophizing

The key to overcoming catastrophizing is to change your mindset. Cognitive-behavioral therapy (CBT) is an effective approach to help individuals recognize and challenge their negative thoughts about pain. By shifting focus from fear and hopelessness to more positive, realistic thoughts, individuals can reduce the psychological burden of pain.

1.5.3 The Influence Of Pain On Quality Of Life

Pain doesn't just affect your body—it also impacts your quality of life. Chronic pain can interfere with daily activities, relationships, work, and social interactions, leading to a diminished sense of well-being. It can be isolating, making you feel disconnected from the world.

Impact On Social Life

Chronic pain can cause people to withdraw socially, fearing that their pain will limit their ability to engage in everyday activities. This isolation can contribute to feelings of loneliness and depression. In some cases, people may even start to feel like a burden to others, which can worsen emotional distress and further reduce their quality of life.

Impact On Work And Productivity

Pain can also affect work performance, leading to missed days, lower productivity, and even job loss. The frustration of not being able to perform as you once did can exacerbate feelings of helplessness and hopelessness.

The Cycle Of Fear And Avoidance

When you experience pain, you may begin to fear certain movements or activities, which can lead to avoidance. This avoidance can result in further deconditioning, weakening muscles, and increasing pain in the long run. Overcoming this fear and re-engaging in physical activity in a controlled manner is essential for improving both physical and mental well-being.

1.5.4 The Role Of Mindfulness And Cognitive-Behavioral Therapy (CBT) In Pain Management

To effectively manage pain, addressing the psychological dimensions is crucial. Mindfulness and **cognitive-behavioral therapy (CBT)** are two powerful techniques that can help you take control of your pain by changing the way you think about it and how you respond to it.

Mindfulness

Mindfulness involves paying attention to the present moment without judgment. By practicing mindfulness, individuals can become more aware of their pain without letting it overwhelm them. Instead of focusing on the pain itself, mindfulness encourages people to focus on their breathing, body, and surroundings, helping them to detach from the pain.

Cognitive-Behavioral Therapy (CBT)

CBT is a structured approach that helps individuals changenegative thought patterns and behavior. In the context of pain management, CBT teaches individuals to reframe negative thoughts about pain and develop healthier coping strategies. This therapy helps reduce pain perception by altering how the brain processes pain signals.

Both mindfulness and CBT have been shown to improve pain tolerance, reduce emotional distress, and help individuals reclaim their lives from the grip of chronic pain.

Conclusion

Understanding The Psychological Dimensions Of Pain

Pain is more than just a physical sensation—it's a complex emotional and psychological experience. By understanding the psychological dimensions of pain, we can develop more comprehensive and effective treatment strategies. Whether it's managing stress, addressing negative thought patterns, or using therapies like CBT and mindfulness, the mind plays a critical role in the manner we experience and manage pain.

Recognizing and addressing the psychological aspects of pain allows us to break free from the cycle of suffering and regain control over our lives.

Chapter 2
Pain And Its Causes

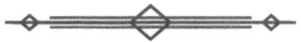

Understanding pain requires delving into its many different forms and origins. While pain is an inevitable part of the human experience, chronic pain, in particular, can be both debilitating and life-altering. This chapter explores the various causes of pain, focusing on common chronic pain conditions. By identifying the underlying sources of pain, we can better understand its mechanisms and work toward more effective treatments.

2.1 Common Chronic Pain Conditions

Chronic pain is not just an occasional nuisance—it's a condition that affects millions of people worldwide, disrupting daily life and often leading to long-term physical, emotional, and psychological consequences. Understanding the most prevalent chronic pain conditions can help both patients and healthcare providers pinpoint the root causes and develop tailored treatment plans.

Here are some of the most common chronic pain conditions:

2.1.1 Osteoarthritis (OA)

Osteoarthritis is one of the most common causes of chronic joint pain, especially in the elderly. It occurs when the cartilage that cushions the ends of your bones wears down over time. While OA can affect any joint, it typically impacts the knees, hips, hands, and spine.

Symptoms

- Stiffness in joints, particularly after periods of inactivity or in the morning
- Pain that worsens with activity and improves with rest
- Swelling, tenderness, and warmth around the joints
- Decreased range of motion

Osteoarthritis can make everyday activities—like walking, climbing stairs, and even grasping objects—difficult or painful. While there is no cure, managing OA through medications, physical therapy, and lifestyle changes can help improve quality of life and reduce symptoms.

2.1.2 Rheumatoid Arthritis (RA)

Rheumatoid arthritis is an autoimmune disorder in which the body's immune system mistakenly attacks the lining of the joints. This leads to inflammation, pain, and eventually joint damage. Unlike osteoarthritis, which typically affects older adults, RA can develop at any age and often manifests earlier in life, especially in women.

Symptoms

- Joint pain, swelling, and stiffness that is usually worse in the morning

- Redness and warmth around affected joints
- Fatigue and malaise
- Symmetrical joint involvement (both sides of the body affected)

In RA, the body's immune response attacks healthy tissue, causing chronic inflammation. Without treatment, RA can lead to permanent joint damage and deformities, but with early intervention and appropriate medication, the condition can be managed effectively.

2.1.3 Fibromyalgia

Fibromyalgia is a disorder characterized by widespread musculoskeletal pain, fatigue, sleep disturbances, and cognitive difficulties. Unlike other pain conditions, fibromyalgia does not cause visible inflammation or physical damage to the tissues. Instead, the pain is believed to result from an abnormal response to pain signals in the brain and nervous system.

Symptoms

- Persistent, widespread pain that affects the muscles, ligaments, and tendons
- Sleep disturbances, often resulting in poor-quality sleep
- Cognitive difficulties (often referred to as "fibro fog"), such as memory issues and trouble concentrating
- Fatigue and depression

Fibromyalgia is notoriously difficult to diagnose, as its symptoms can overlap with those of other conditions. However, a combination of medications, lifestyle changes, physical therapy, and stress management techniques can provide relief and help individuals manage their symptoms.

2.1.4 Chronic Back Pain

Chronic back pain is one of the most common and most debilitating types of chronic pain, affecting individuals of all ages. It can result from various causes, including injuries, degenerative diseases, and poor posture. Chronic back pain can significantly affect mobility and quality of life, often causing disability and preventing people from participating in everyday activities.

Symptoms

- Persistent lower back pain that lasts for weeks or months
- Pain that radiates down the legs (sciatica)
- Limited mobility and difficulty bending or twisting
- Muscle spasms and stiffness

Chronic back pain may be due to herniated discs, spinal stenosis, osteoarthritis, or muscle strains. Treatment options range from physical therapy and medications to more invasive treatments like injections or surgery, depending on the severity of the condition.

2.1.5 Migraines And Tension Headaches

Headaches, particularly migraines and tension headaches, are common sources of chronic pain that can be incredibly debilitating. While many people experience occasional headaches, chronic headaches can occur multiple times a week, significantly affecting a person's ability to function normally.

Migraines

Migraines are intense, throbbing headaches that are often accompanied by other symptoms such as nausea, vomiting, and sensitivity to light or sound. Migraines can last for hours or even days, severely affecting daily life. They are often triggered by factors such as stress, hormonal changes, certain foods, or environmental factors.

Tension Headaches

Tension headaches, while typically less severe than migraines, are the most common type of headache. They are characterized by a constant, dull pain or pressure around the head, often associated with muscle tension in the neck and shoulders.

Chronic migraines and tension headaches can lead to significant distress and discomfort, but there are effective treatments, including medications, lifestyle modifications, and stress management techniques, that can help reduce the frequency and severity of these headaches.

2.1.6 Neuropathic Pain

Damage or dysfunction of the nerves themselves, not tissue injury, causes neuropathic pain. Conditions such as diabetes, shingles, and multiple sclerosis can cause nerve damage that leads to chronic pain. Neuropathic pain can be particularly challenging to treat because it often involves abnormal pain signaling from the nerves, leading to sensations of burning, tingling, or shooting pain.

Symptoms

- Sharp, stabbing pain
- Numbness or tingling sensations
- Sensitivity to touch or temperature changes
- Shooting pain or electric shock-like sensations

Neuropathic pain is often treated with medications that target nerve function, such as anticonvulsants, antidepressants, or topical treatments. Physical therapy and nerve blocks may also be beneficial in managing symptoms.

Conclusion

Chronic pain conditions vary widely in terms of causes, symptoms, and treatments. From the degenerative nature of osteoarthritis to the complex, mysterious pain of fibromyalgia, these conditions are diverse, affecting people's lives in different ways. However, understanding the causes and mechanisms behind these conditions allows healthcare providers to offer better, more targeted treatments.

Whether through physical therapy, medication, or lifestyle changes, individuals living with chronic pain can find ways to manage their symptoms and improve their quality of life. The next step is not just about addressing the physical aspect of pain but understanding its broader implications on mental and emotional well-being, which we will explore in the following chapter

2.2 Lifestyle and Environmental Factors

Chronic pain doesn't just arise from injuries, medical conditions, or genetic factors; lifestyle choices and environmental influences also play a significant role in how pain develops, manifests, and persists. Pain is a complex experience that involves the interplay of physical, psychological, and environmental factors. How we live, what we eat, and the world around us can either exacerbate or help alleviate chronic pain. In this section, we explore the impact of lifestyle and environmental factors on chronic pain and the crucial role they play in its management and prevention.

2.2.1 The Impact Of Diet On Chronic Pain

What we eat can directly affect inflammation, joint health, and overall pain levels. Certain foods may trigger inflammation, while others can help reduce it. Understanding how diet influences pain and how making mindful food choices can ease discomfort is essential for those dealing with chronic pain.

Pro-Inflammatory Vs. Anti-Inflammatory Foods

The foods we eat can either promote inflammation, which contributes to pain, or fight it. Pro-inflammatory foods—

such as refined sugars, trans fats, and highly processed foods—can increase inflammation in the body, leading to exacerbated pain, particularly in conditions like osteoarthritis and rheumatoid arthritis. On the other hand, anti-inflammatory foods, such as fruits, vegetables, whole grains, and omega-3-rich foods like fish and flaxseeds, have the potential to reduce inflammation and provide relief from chronic pain.

Common Pain-Exacerbating Foods

- Processed meats (such as bacon and sausages)
- Refined sugars and baked goods
- Fried foods and trans fats
- Dairy (in some individuals with sensitivities)

Pain-Relieving Foods

- Fatty fish (salmon, mackerel, sardines)
- Berries (rich in antioxidants)
- Leafy greens (spinach, kale)
- Nuts (almonds, walnuts)
- Turmeric and ginger (natural anti-inflammatory agents)

Dietary changes can significantly reduce the level of pain for individuals suffering from chronic inflammatory conditions. In some cases, food sensitivity testing and an elimination diet may be necessary to identify specific triggers that aggravate pain.

2.2.2 Exercise: A Double-Edged Sword

Exercise is often recommended as part of a pain management plan, but it's a complex relationship. While regular physical activity can strengthen muscles, improve flexibility, and reduce pain over time, improper or excessive exercise can exacerbate pain, especially in individuals with conditions like osteoarthritis or fibromyalgia.

The Right Type of Exercise

Exercise must be tailored to an individual's condition and needs. Gentle exercises such as swimming, yoga, or walking can help improve mobility and reduce stiffness, while high-impact activities like running or heavy lifting may worsen joint pain or muscle strains. Strength training can be particularly beneficial for those with arthritis, as it helps support the joints and improves overall function.

The Role of Stretching and Mobility Work

Stretching exercises can improve joint range of motion and reduce muscle tension, two key contributors to pain. Regular flexibility training, combined with strengthening exercises, can help prevent further injury and decrease chronic pain over time.

However, it's essential to listen to your body—pushing through intense pain during exercise may lead to injury or exacerbate existing pain. A personalized, gradual approach to exercise is key to preventing flare-ups and improving overall pain management.

2.2.3 Sleep and Chronic Pain

Sleep plays a crucial role in pain management and recovery. Chronic pain can disrupt sleep, leading to a vicious cycle of pain, poor sleep, and fatigue. Inadequate sleep can heighten the perception of pain, reduce pain tolerance, and make it harder for the body to heal.

The Connection Between Sleep and Pain

When you don't get enough sleep, the body's ability to recover from physical exertion and injury is hindered. During sleep, the body produces growth hormones and other chemicals that promote healing, tissue repair, and immune function. Lack of restorative sleep can also increase inflammation and heighten pain sensitivity.

People with chronic pain often experience disturbed sleep patterns, whether from pain-related discomfort or conditions like insomnia, sleep apnea, or restless leg syndrome. In turn, poor sleep worsens pain, creating a cycle that can be difficult to break.

Improving Sleep Hygiene

Practices that promote better sleep include:

- Creating a calming bedtime routine (e.g, reading, meditating, taking a warm bath)
- Keeping a consistent sleep schedule
- Using comfortable pillows and mattresses that support joint health
- Limiting screen time before bed

- Avoiding caffeine and heavy meals close to bedtime

In some cases, pain management interventions like nerve blocks, medications, or physical therapy can improve sleep quality and break the pain-sleep cycle.

2.2.4 Stress and Its Role In Pain

Stress is a significant environmental factor that can make chronic pain worse. The body's stress response can activate the sympathetic nervous system, releasing cortisol, adrenaline, and other chemicals that trigger inflammation, muscle tension, and increased pain sensitivity. Stress also affects pain perception, making individuals more sensitive to discomfort and less resilient in managing their pain.

Psychological Stress and Pain Amplification

Emotional stress, anxiety, and depression can intensify physical pain. In conditions like fibromyalgia or chronic back pain, stress often leads to muscle spasms, tension, and heightened pain sensitivity. Moreover, stress can lead to poor coping strategies such as overexertion, unhealthy eating, or insufficient sleep, which only serve to exacerbate pain.

Stress-Reduction Techniques

Techniques that reduce stress and promote relaxation can help break this cycle.

- Meditation and mindfulness practices
- Deep breathing exercises

- Progressive muscle relaxation
- Cognitive-behavioral therapy (CBT)
- Biofeedback

These techniques help calm the nervous system, reduce muscle tension, and improve overall well-being, providing significant relief for those living with chronic pain.

2.2.5 The Influence of Environmental Factors

Environmental factors such as climate, living conditions, and exposure to toxins or pollutants can also contribute to or worsen chronic pain. For example, people with arthritis often report an increase in pain during cold or humid weather, while environmental stressors like noise pollution or poor air quality can also aggravate symptoms.

Weather And Pain Sensitivity

Many individuals with chronic pain conditions report increased pain during cold, damp, or stormy weather. The exact reasons for this are still not entirely clear, but it is believed that barometric pressure changes affect joint tissues, making them stiffer and more prone to pain.

Toxin Exposure And Pain

Exposure to environmental toxins, such as pesticides or chemicals in household cleaning products, may lead to inflammation and worsen pain conditions. Additionally, individuals with respiratory conditions like asthma may experience increased pain due to poor air quality or high levels of pollution in their environment.

In some cases, individuals may need to make environmental adjustments, such as using air purifiers, moving to a warmer climate, or avoiding prolonged exposure to environmental stressors.

Conclusion

The environment and lifestyle choices play a crucial role in managing and alleviating chronic pain. From the foods we eat to how we move our bodies, and from our stress levels to our sleep habits, these factors can either exacerbate or reduce the intensity of chronic pain. By adopting healthy lifestyle habits, such as a balanced diet, regular exercise, adequate sleep, stress management, and environmental awareness, individuals can take control of their pain and improve their quality of life

2.3 How Poor Posture Causes Pain

Posture, though often overlooked, plays a critical role in how the body functions and pain manifests. Poor posture, whether from sitting at a desk for hours, slouching, or improper body mechanics during physical activity, can lead to a cascade of issues that result in chronic pain. In this section, we explore how poor posture affects the body and contributes to various types of pain, particularly in the spine, neck, shoulders, and lower back.

2.3.1 The Mechanisms of Posture

Posture refers to the alignment and positioning of the body while standing, sitting, or moving. When we adopt a neutral, well-aligned posture, the bones, muscles, and joints are all in their optimal positions, and the body works efficiently. However, when we slouch or hunch over, we place excess strain on certain muscles, ligaments, and joints, leading to misalignment and discomfort.

Poor posture may arise from a number of factors, such as prolonged sitting, improper ergonomics, or muscle imbalances. It is often unnoticed until pain sets in, but over time, poor posture can lead to significant long-term health issues.

2.3.2 Common Areas Affected By Poor Posture

The spine, being the central structure of the body, is the most impacted by poor posture. When we slouch or lean forward, the natural curve of the spine is disrupted, leading to muscle strain, tension, and misalignment in the vertebrae.

Neck And Shoulders

Forward head posture, where the head juts out in front of the body instead of being aligned with the spine, is a common result of poor posture. This misalignment places a significant burden on the neck and shoulder muscles, leading to stiffness, headaches, and even chronic neck pain. Over time, this can contribute to conditions like cervical spondylosis or muscle imbalances that exacerbate pain.

Lower Back

Slouching, particularly when sitting for long periods, places additional pressure on the lumbar spine (lower back), which can lead to muscle fatigue, disc compression, and lower back pain. Poor posture while standing, such as excessive arching or leaning forward, can also lead to lower back strain and conditions like sciatica.

Hips And Pelvis

When we sit with a poor posture, such as slouching or leaning to one side, it can disrupt the alignment of the pelvis and hips. Over time, this misalignment can lead to hip pain, pelvic discomfort, and even complications like hip bursitis or sacroiliac joint pain.

2.3.3 The Long-Term Effects of Poor Posture

Over time, poor posture can lead to various of chronic pain conditions as muscles and ligaments become strained and imbalanced. These issues may become more pronounced with age as the body's ability to recover from these misalignments diminishes.

Degenerative Disc Disease

Chronic poor posture can accelerate wear and tear on the spinal discs, leading to degenerative disc disease. Misalignment causes uneven pressure on the discs, resulting in disc herniation, bulging discs, or even disc rupture, all of which contribute to ongoing back and neck pain.

Muscle Imbalances

When one part of the body is overworked due to poor posture, other muscles may weaken or become stretched out. This imbalance can create a domino effect, causing pain to spread to other areas of the body. For example, tight chest muscles from slouching may lead to upper back pain, while weak abdominal muscles from improper posture may contribute to lower back issues.

2.3.4 Correcting Posture For Pain Relief

The good news is that poor posture can be corrected with awareness, physical therapy, and consistent practice. Correcting posture may not only relieve current pain but can prevent future pain and improve overall quality of life.

Posture Awareness

The first step in improving posture is developing an awareness of how we sit, stand, and move. Small adjustments, such as sitting with both feet flat on the floor, keeping the shoulders back, and aligning the ears with the shoulders, can make a big difference.

Ergonomic Adjustments

Workspaces should be set up to promote good posture. This includes using chairs that support the lower back, keeping the computer monitor at eye level, and ensuring the desk height encourages a neutral wrist position. Taking regular breaks from sitting and incorporating movement throughout the day also helps reduce strain.

Exercise And Stretching

Strengthening exercises, particularly for the core and back muscles, can help support good posture and alleviate pain. Stretching exercises, such as yoga, can improve flexibility and relieve tension caused by poor posture. Regular physical activity helps maintain good alignment and prevent imbalances.

Conclusion

Poor posture is a widespread but often preventable cause of chronic pain. By paying attention to body mechanics, making ergonomic adjustments, and practicing posture-correcting exercises, individuals can alleviate pain and reduce the risk of developing long-term pain conditions. Simple changes in how we sit, stand, and move can have a profound impact on our overall well-being and quality of life.

2.4 Hormonal Impact on Pain In Women

Hormones are vital chemical messengers that regulate various bodily functions, including pain perception. In women, hormonal fluctuations related to the menstrual cycle, pregnancy, and menopause can significantly impact pain intensity, sensitivity, and tolerance. In this section, we will explore how hormonal changes contribute to pain, particularly in women, and how to manage these fluctuations.

2.4.1 Menstrual Cycle And Pain

The menstrual cycle, which involves regular hormonal changes, can influence pain sensitivity in women. Many women experience discomfort before and during menstruation, often referred to as dysmenorrhea. These pains are typically caused by changes in the hormone prostaglandin, which triggers uterine contractions, leading to cramping and lower back pain.

Prostaglandins And Pain Sensitivity

Prostaglandins are chemicals released during the menstrual cycle that help the uterus contract to shed its lining. High levels of prostaglandins can cause stronger contractions, leading to more intense cramps and pain. In some women, the pain can be debilitating, interfering with daily activities, and requiring medical treatment.

Managing Menstrual Pain

Nonsteroidal anti-inflammatory drugs (NSAIDs), such as ibuprofen, are commonly used to reduce prostaglandin production and alleviate menstrual pain. Additionally, other treatments such as heat therapy, exercise, or acupuncture may also help relieve discomfort.

2.4.2 Pregnancy and Pain Sensitivity

Pregnancy is another time when hormonal changes can increase pain sensitivity. During pregnancy, the body undergoes a series of adjustments to accommodate the growing fetus, leading to pain in various areas.

Hormonal Relaxation and Joint Pain

As pregnancy progresses, the hormone relaxin is released, which loosens the ligaments and joints to prepare for childbirth. While this helps with delivery, it can also cause instability and discomfort, particularly in the hips, pelvis, and lower back.

Managing Pregnancy-Related Pain

Gentle exercises, physical therapy, and proper posture can help manage pregnancy-related pain. Prenatal massage and the use of a maternity support belt can also provide relief.

2.4.3 Menopause and Chronic Pain

Menopause, which marks the end of a woman's reproductive years, brings about significant hormonal shifts that can impact pain sensitivity. The decline in estrogen levels can affect the musculoskeletal system, leading to an increased risk of joint pain, muscle stiffness, and conditions like osteoarthritis.

Estrogen's Role in Pain Perception

Estrogen plays a role in regulating pain pathways in the body. When estrogen levels drop during menopause, women may experience increased sensitivity to pain, particularly in the joints and muscles. Hot flashes, another common symptom of menopause, can also contribute to discomfort and exacerbate pain.

Managing Menopausal Pain

Hormone replacement therapy (HRT) can be an effective treatment for some women to manage menopausal symptoms, including pain. Additionally, regular exercise, maintaining a healthy weight, and dietary adjustments can help reduce inflammation and improve overall pain management.

2.4.4 Hormonal Migraines

Some women experience migraines that are triggered or worsened by hormonal changes. These hormonal migraines are often linked to fluctuations in estrogen levels, particularly around menstruation, pregnancy, and menopause. Migraines can be debilitating, causing throbbing head pain, nausea, and sensitivity to light and sound.

Managing Hormonal Migraines

Migraine prevention strategies include identifying triggers, using medications like triptans, and incorporating lifestyle changes such as adequate sleep, hydration, and avoiding stress.

2.4.5 Hormonal Impact on Fibromyalgia And Chronic Pain Conditions

Women are more likely to develop fibromyalgia, a condition characterized by widespread musculoskeletal pain, and hormonal changes may play a role in its development. Fluctuating estrogen and progesterone levels may affect the way the brain processes pain signals, leading to increased pain sensitivity in women with fibromyalgia.

Conclusion

Hormonal changes significantly influence how women experience pain. From menstrual cramps to pregnancy-related discomfort and the pain associated with menopause, understanding the hormonal impact on pain is key to effective management. A combination of medical treatments, lifestyle changes, and self-care practices can help women navigate these hormonal fluctuations and alleviate pain.

2.5 Pain in The Elderly: Unique Challenges

As individuals age, the body undergoes a series of changes that can lead to chronic pain. These changes, both physical and neurological, contribute to a heightened vulnerability to conditions that cause pain, such as arthritis, osteoporosis, and neuropathy. Chronic pain in the elderly is often misunderstood, as it can manifest differently and may be complicated by other health conditions. In this section, we will explore the unique challenges faced by older adults in managing pain and the ways that healthcare providers can help improve their quality of life.

2.5.1 The Aging Body and Pain Sensitivity

As people age, the body's ability to repair tissues and regenerate cells decreases. This can lead to slower healing times and increased susceptibility to pain. One of the most significant changes is the degradation of cartilage in the joints, leading to osteoarthritis, a common source of joint pain in the elderly.

Reduced Muscle Mass and Bone Density

With age, muscle mass tends to decrease, and bones become weaker, a condition known as sarcopenia and osteoporosis. These changes increase the risk of falls, fractures, and general muscle and joint pain. The decreased strength and flexibility in muscles and joints can make simple movements painful, contributing to a cycle of inactivity, which only worsens the condition.

Slower Nervous System Response

As the nervous system ages, it becomes less efficient at transmitting signals, including those related to pain. This can lead to an altered pain perception. In some cases, the elderly may feel pain more intensely due to heightened sensitivity in the nervous system. On the other hand, some elderly individuals may have a diminished response to pain, which can delay diagnosis and treatment of underlying health issues.

2.5.2 Chronic Pain Conditions Common in The Elderly

Chronic pain is prevalent in older adults, and the conditions that cause it can significantly impact daily living. Some of the most common conditions that contribute to pain in the elderly include:

Osteoarthritis (OA)

Osteoarthritis is a degenerative joint disease that causes the cartilage in the joints to break down, leading to pain, stiffness, and swelling. OA is particularly common in the knees, hips, and hands and can severely limit mobility. As cartilage wears away, bones can rub together, intensifying the pain.

Osteoporosis And Fractures

Osteoporosis causes bones to become brittle and fragile, increasing the risk of fractures even from minor falls or movements. Spinal fractures are particularly common in the elderly, leading to back pain and often resulting in a hunched posture. These fractures can contribute to long-term, debilitating pain that reduces the elderly person's independence and mobility.

Peripheral Neuropathy

This condition, which results from damage to the peripheral nerves, is common in older adults, particularly those with diabetes. It can cause numbness, tingling, and burning sensations, often in the feet and hands. In some cases, peripheral neuropathy can result in severe pain that interferes with daily activities, sleep, and overall quality of life.

Rheumatoid Arthritis (RA)

Unlike osteoarthritis, rheumatoid arthritis is an autoimmune condition where the immune system mistakenly attacks healthy joints. RA often causes inflammation, severe pain, and stiffness, particularly in the hands, wrists, and knees. The elderly may experience heightened symptoms and increased difficulty in managing these flare-ups.

Cancer Pain

Cancer is another common cause of chronic pain in older adults. The pain may be caused by the tumour pressing on surrounding tissues or by treatments such as chemotherapy and radiation. Cancer pain is often complex and requires a multi-disciplinary approach to ensure proper management.

2.5.3 Multimorbidity and Pain Management

Many elderly individuals suffer from multiple chronic conditions simultaneously, a phenomenon known as multimorbidity. This complicates pain management, as the treatment of one condition may exacerbate another. For example, nonsteroidal anti-inflammatory drugs (NSAIDs) used to treat arthritis can negatively impact kidney function, particularly in elderly patients with pre-existing kidney disease.

Polypharmacy

Elderly individuals often take multiple medications to manage their various health conditions. This increases the risk of drug interactions, side effects, and potential overmedication. Balancing pain relief while minimizing the risks of polypharmacy is a significant challenge for healthcare providers. Many elderly patients are also hesitant to use strong pain medications, such as opioids, due to concerns about addiction or side effects.

Cognitive Decline and Pain

Cognitive decline, including conditions like dementia, can make it difficult for elderly individuals to communicate their pain effectively. They may not be able to articulate their discomfort, leading to under reporting of pain and delayed treatment. Caregivers must be attentive to non-verbal cues, such as changes in behavior or increased agitation, which can indicate pain in those with cognitive impairments.

2.5.4 Psychological Factors in Chronic Pain

Chronic pain in the elderly is often associated with emotional and psychological challenges. The burden of living with ongoing pain can lead to depression, anxiety, and a reduced sense of well-being. In turn, these psychological issues can make pain management even more challenging, creating a cycle of pain and emotional distress.

Depression And Pain Sensitivity

Depression is common among elderly individuals living with chronic pain. It can alter pain perception, making individuals more sensitive to discomfort. Depression can also result in a lack of motivation to engage in physical therapy or exercise, which further exacerbates pain and disability.

Anxiety And Fear Of Movement

Elderly patients with chronic pain may develop an exaggerated fear of movement (kinesiophobia), particularly after experiencing a fall or injury. This fear can lead to physical deconditioning, as they may avoid activity to prevent pain or injury. This can increase their vulnerability to further pain and disability, reinforcing the cycle.

2.5.5 Effective Pain Management Strategies For The Elderly

Effective pain management in the elderly requires a comprehensive, multi-faceted approach. Healthcare providers need to consider not just the physical aspects of pain but also the emotional and psychological challenges. Below are some key strategies:

Physical Therapy And Exercise

Physical therapy is one of the most effective ways to manage pain in the elderly. Gentle exercises, stretching routines, and strengthening programs can help improve mobility, reduce stiffness, and alleviate pain. Regular physical activity also helps maintain bone density, muscle strength, and joint flexibility.

Non-Pharmacological Interventions

In addition to medications, non-pharmacological treatments such as acupuncture, massage therapy, heat and cold applications, and cognitive behavioral therapy (CBT) can provide significant pain relief. These treatments are particularly beneficial for elderly individuals who may not tolerate medications well.

Medications And Pain Relief

While medication should be prescribed carefully, analgesics such as acetaminophen and topical pain relievers can be helpful in managing mild to moderate pain. For more severe pain, opioids or stronger medications may be necessary, but they should be used with caution. Regular monitoring for side effects and potential drug interactions is essential.

Supportive Care and Lifestyle Modifications

Assisting the elderly with maintaining a supportive environment, such as grab bars, walkers, and adaptive devices, can reduce the strain on their bodies and prevent further injury. Nutritional counselling and managing comorbidities, such as diabetes or hypertension, are also essential in supporting pain management and overall well-being.

Conclusion

Pain in the elderly presents unique challenges, from physical degeneration and chronic conditions to psychological factors that complicate treatment. However, with a comprehensive and tailored approach, healthcare providers can help elderly individuals manage their pain and improve their quality of life. The key lies in understanding the multifaceted nature of pain in this demographic and addressing both the physical and emotional components to provide effective and compassionate care.

Chapter 3
Innovations In Pain Relief

3.1 Cutting-Edge Technology in Pain Management

Pain management has evolved dramatically over the years, with technological advancements playing a key role in improving how pain is diagnosed, treated, and managed. In this chapter, we explore the innovative technologies that are transforming pain relief, offering patients new hope and more effective solutions. From advanced diagnostic tools to groundbreaking treatment techniques, these technologies are shaping the future of pain management.

3.1.1 Medical Imaging Advancements

One of the most significant innovations in pain management is the advancement in medical imaging techniques. High-resolution imaging technologies allow healthcare providers to pinpoint the exact source of pain with greater accuracy. Tools such as **MRI (Magnetic Resonance Imaging)**, **CT scans (Computed Tomography)**, and **PET scans (Positron Emission Tomography)** enable doctors to observe internal structures in real time, providing a clearer understanding of conditions such as spinal disc herniation, joint inflammation, and nerve damage.

- **Functional MRI (fMRI):** fMRI is an innovative imaging technique that not only helps diagnose structural issues but also measures brain activity in response to pain. This has opened new doors in understanding how pain is processed in the brain, leading to more targeted and effective treatments.

- **Thermal Imaging:** Thermal imaging systems are being used to assess changes in temperature that indicate inflammation or abnormal tissue growth. These systems offer a non-invasive, real-time way to monitor areas of pain and track progress in pain treatment.

By utilizing these imaging technologies, pain physicians can identify the exact source of a patient's pain, which leads to more accurate diagnoses and personalized treatment plans.

3.1.2 Neuromodulation Techniques

Neuromodulation refers to the use of technology to alter nerve activity in the body. This approach is particularly effective in managing chronic pain, especially for conditions where traditional methods have failed. These methods target the nervous system to alleviate pain, providing relief for conditions such as neuropathic pain, fibromyalgia, and complex regional pain syndrome (CRPS).

- **Spinal Cord Stimulation (SCS):** Spinal cord stimulators are implanted devices that deliver electrical impulses to the spinal cord, effectively "masking" pain signals before they reach the brain. This method has proven highly effective for patients with chronic back pain and leg pain.

- **Peripheral Nerve Stimulation (PNS)**: PNS involves the use of electrical impulses delivered to specific peripheral nerves to reduce pain. This technique is often used for conditions like post-surgical pain, migraines, and phantom limb pain.

- **Transcranial Magnetic Stimulation (TMS)**: TMS is a non-invasive treatment that uses magnetic fields to stimulate nerve cells in the brain. This method has shown promise in treating chronic pain, especially for conditions like fibromyalgia and depression-associated pain.

Neuromodulation offers a non-drug approach to pain relief, reducing the reliance on opioids and other pain medications while also improving the quality of life for many patients.

3.1.3 Regenerative Medicine: Stem Cells and Platelet-Rich Plasma (PRP)

Regenerative medicine has emerged as a groundbreaking field with great promise for pain relief, especially for conditions involving tissue damage, degeneration, or inflammation. These innovative therapies stimulate the body's natural healing processes and repair damaged tissues, offering long-term relief.

- **Stem Cell Therapy**: Stem cells are undifferentiated cells capable of developing into various types of tissues. In pain management, stem cells are used to regenerate damaged cartilage, bones, and muscles, particularly in the cases of osteoarthritis or tendon injuries. By injecting stem cells directly into the damaged tissue, it becomes possible to accelerate the healing process and reduce pain.

- **Platelet-Rich Plasma (PRP) Therapy**: PRP therapy involves drawing a patient's blood, processing it to concentrate the platelets, and injecting it back into the area of injury or pain. The growth factors in PRP help to stimulate tissue repair, reduce inflammation, and promote healing. PRP therapy is widely used in musculoskeletal pain, including joint and tendon issues.

Both stem cell and PRP therapies have the potential to provide lasting pain relief and restore functionality, allowing patients to return to their daily activities without the need for surgery or long-term medication use.

3.1.4 Laser Therapy: Low-Level Laser Therapy (LLLT)

Low-Level Laser Therapy (LLLT), also known as cold laser therapy, is a non-invasive treatment that uses specific wavelengths of light to stimulate cellular repair and reduce inflammation. LLLT has become an increasingly popular option for treating musculoskeletal pain, soft tissue injuries, and even nerve pain.

- **Mechanism Of Action:** LLLT works by penetrating the skin and reaching the deeper layers of tissue, where it stimulates mitochondrial function, increases blood flow, and reduces oxidative stress. These effects accelerate the body's natural healing processes and promote pain relief.

- **Conditions Treated:** LLLT is used to treat a variety of pain conditions, including arthritis, tendinitis, sprains, and carpal tunnel syndrome. It is also beneficial for healing wounds and injuries, particularly in athletes.

Unlike traditional laser treatments that use high heat to remove tissue, LLLT uses low intensity to promote healing without causing any harm to the surrounding tissues, making it a safe and effective treatment option.

3.1.5 Artificial Intelligence and Pain Management

Pain management practices are increasingly integrating artificial intelligence (AI) to help doctors make more accurate diagnoses, predict treatment outcomes, and optimize treatment plans. AI algorithms can analyse vast amounts of data, including patient health records, imaging results, and even genetic information, to provide personalized pain management strategies.

- **Predictive Analytics**: AI can analyse patient data to predict pain progression and the likelihood of developing chronic pain. This helps doctors intervene early and adjust treatment plans to prevent pain from becoming long-term or debilitating.

- **Robot-Assisted Surgery**: In some cases, AI-powered robotic systems are used to assist in surgeries, such as joint replacements, where precision is critical. These systems help minimize human error and speed up recovery times, leading to less pain post-surgery.

AI is also being explored for virtual health assistants that can monitor patients' symptoms in real time and provide guidance on pain management strategies, further empowering patients to take control of their pain.

Conclusion

The landscape of pain management is rapidly changing thanks to technological innovations. From advanced imaging techniques that provide clearer diagnoses to cutting-edge treatments like neuromodulation and regenerative medicine, these developments offer patients new opportunities for effective and lasting pain relief. As technology continues to evolve, the potential for improved pain management expands, bringing hope to millions of people living with chronic pain. Future advancements are paving the way for more effective pain control and improved quality of life for patients.

3.2 Stem Cells and Regenerative Medicine

Stem cell therapy and regenerative medicine are revolutionizing the field of pain management by offering innovative solutions for treating conditions that were previously thought to require surgery or long-term medication. These treatments harness the body's natural ability to heal itself, repairing damaged tissues and alleviating pain without invasive procedures.

3.2.1 Stem Cell Therapy: Healing from Within

Stem cells have the unique ability to regenerate damaged tissues and promote healing, which makes them invaluable in treating chronic pain caused by conditions such as osteoarthritis, tendonitis, and degenerative disc disease. Stem cell therapy works by injecting concentrated stem cells directly into the area of injury or damage, stimulating tissue regeneration and reducing inflammation.

- **Types Of Stem Cells Used in Pain Treatment:**
    - **Autologous Stem Cells:** These are stem cells harvested from the patient's own body, typically from bone marrow or adipose (fat) tissue. Using the patient's cells minimize the risk of rejection and side effects.
    - **Allogenic Stem Cells:** These stem cells are sourced from a donor and are used when the patient's stem cells are not suitable for treatment. These stem cells undergo rigorous testing to ensure their safety and effectiveness.
- **Conditions Treated with Stem Cells:** Stem cell therapy is used to treat a variety of painful conditions, including:
    - **Osteoarthritis:** Stem cells can help regenerate cartilage and reduce inflammation

in joints affected by arthritis. Tendon Injuries: Stem cells facilitate the healing of torn or damaged tendons, thereby reducing pain and restoring function.

- **Spinal Disc Degeneration:** Stem cells can help regenerate spinal discs, which may relieve chronic back and neck pain.

Stem cell therapy offers hope for patients who suffer from chronic pain and have exhausted other treatment options. As research in this field continues to grow, it's expected that stem cell treatments will become even more effective and accessible.

3.2.2 Platelet-Rich Plasma (PRP) Therapy: Harnessing the Power of Platelets

Platelet-rich plasma (PRP) therapy is another groundbreaking form of regenerative medicine that utilizes the body's platelets to promote healing and reduce pain. Platelets, which are blood cells that help with clotting, also contain growth factors that play a crucial role in tissue repair.

- **How PRP Therapy Works:** In PRP therapy, a patient's blood is drawn and processed to concentrate the platelets. This platelet-rich plasma is then injected into the area of injury or pain, stimulating tissue regeneration, reducing inflammation, and accelerating healing.

- **Conditions Treated With PRP**: PRP therapy is effective for treating conditions such as:

- **Chronic Tendon Injuries**: Tendonitis and tendon tears, common in athletes, can benefit from PRP, which accelerates healing and reduces pain.

- **Osteoarthritis**: PRP can help regenerate cartilage in the joints and reduce inflammation, providing relief for patients with arthritis.

- **Soft Tissue Injuries**: PRP is also used to treat ligament and muscle injuries, where it can promote faster healing and restore functionality.

PRP therapy is often used in conjunction with stem cell therapy to enhance the healing process. It offers a minimally invasive alternative to surgery, making it an attractive option for many patients.

3.2.3 The Future of Regenerative Medicine

The future of stem cells and regenerative medicine holds great promise for pain management. Researchers are exploring new ways to enhance the effectiveness of stem cell treatments, including the development of **genetically modified stem cells**, which could potentially treat a wider range of conditions.

- **Gene Editing in Regenerative Medicine:** The use of CRISPR technology and other gene-editing tools is allowing scientists to modify stem cells to better target specific areas of damage, enhancing the healing process and reducing the need for repeated treatments.

- **Bioprinting:** Another exciting development in regenerative medicine is bioprinting, which involves printing tissues and even organs using a 3D printer. In the future, bio-printed tissues could be used to replace damaged or worn-out tissues in the body, offering a permanent solution to pain caused by injuries or degenerative conditions.

As regenerative medicine continues to evolve, it will undoubtedly offer more patients the possibility of pain relief and healing without the need for invasive surgeries or long-term drug use.

3.3 The Future of Non-Surgical Techniques

Non-surgical techniques are transforming the field of pain management by providing patients with effective treatments that require little to no recovery time. These approaches offer a less invasive alternative to traditional surgery, helping to manage and alleviate pain in a variety of conditions.

3.3.1 Minimally Invasive Procedures

Minimally invasive procedures have been a game-changer in pain management. These procedures involve small incisions or no incisions at all, using advanced imaging techniques such as fluoroscopy or ultrasound to guide the doctor in performing the treatment. Some of the most common minimally invasive procedures include:

- **Facet Joint Injections:** These injections target the small joints in the spine, often providing relief from lower back and neck pain caused by arthritis or disc degeneration.

- **Radiofrequency Ablation (RFA)**: RFA involves using heat to destroy nerve tissue responsible for transmitting pain signals, providing long-lasting relief for patients with chronic pain conditions like arthritis or sciatica.

- **Epidural Steroid Injections**: These injections deliver steroids directly to the epidural space around the spine, reducing inflammation and providing relief for conditions such as herniated discs or spinal stenosis.

These minimally invasive procedures are performed on an outpatient basis, allowing patients to return to their daily activities quickly. They are particularly useful for patients who are not candidates for surgery or those who want to avoid it.

3.3.2 Targeted Pain Relief with Infusion Therapy

Infusion therapy involves the administration of medications directly into the bloodstream through an intravenous (IV) line. This allows for faster and more targeted pain relief compared to oral medications. It is often used for patients with chronic pain conditions who do not respond to traditional pain management methods.

- **Intravenous Ketamine Infusion:** Ketamine is an anesthetic that has shown promise in treating severe chronic pain, especially for conditions such as fibromyalgia, complex regional pain syndrome (CRPS), and neuropathic pain.

- **IV Lidocaine Therapy:** Lidocaine is a local anesthetic that can be administered intravenously to reduce pain and inflammation, particularly for patients with conditions like post-surgical pain or severe nerve pain.

Infusion therapies offer a non-surgical alternative to managing chronic pain, with the added benefit of minimal side effects and faster results.

3.3.3 The Role of Physical Therapy And Exercise

Physical therapy and exercise are essential components of non-surgical pain relief. Physical therapists work with patients to develop personalized exercise programs that help strengthen muscles, improve flexibility, and reduce pain. These therapies are particularly effective for patients with musculoskeletal pain, such as back pain, joint pain, and arthritis.

- **Therapeutic Exercises:** Strengthening exercises can help support weakened muscles around painful joints, reducing strain and alleviating pain. Stretching exercises improve flexibility and reduce stiffness, while aerobic exercises promote overall physical health and well-being.

- **Aquatic Therapy:** Aquatic therapy involves exercises performed in a pool, using the buoyancy of the water to reduce pressure on the joints and provide relief for patients with arthritis or joint pain.

As technology continues to advance, more physical therapy options are becoming available, including virtual therapy sessions and at-home exercise programs, allowing patients to manage their pain more effectively.

3.4 Artificial Intelligence in Diagnostics

Artificial intelligence (AI) is revolutionizing the field of pain management by improving diagnostic accuracy and helping doctors make more informed treatment decisions. AI technologies are being used to analyze vast amounts of medical data, including imaging results, patient histories, and genetic information, to provide personalized treatment plans.

3.4.1 AI In Medical Imaging

One of the most significant ways AI is transforming pain management is through its application in medical imaging. AI-powered systems can analyze X-rays, MRIs, CT scans, and other imaging results with incredible accuracy, detecting even the smallest abnormalities that might be missed by the human eye. These systems are capable of identifying issues such as nerve compression, joint degeneration, and soft tissue damage, enabling doctors to make quicker and more accurate diagnoses.

- **Automated Image Interpretation:** AI algorithms can now automatically interpret medical images, providing doctors with detailed reports and helping them identify the root cause of a patient's pain.

- **Predictive Analytics:** AI can also predict the progression of a condition based on imaging data, helping doctors plan appropriate interventions before the condition worsens.

AI-powered imaging tools are making the diagnostic process faster, more accurate, and more efficient, ultimately leading to better outcomes for patients.

3.4.2 AI In Personalized Treatment Plans

AI's ability to analyze large amounts of patient data allows it to create personalized treatment plans tailored to each individual's unique needs. By considering factors such as genetics, lifestyle, and response to previous treatments, AI can recommend the most effective therapies for managing pain.

- **Predictive Analytics for Pain Progression:** AI can predict how a patient's pain will progress over time, helping doctors proactively manage the condition and avoid flare-ups or complications.

- **Treatment Optimization:** AI can optimize treatment plans by continuously analyzing a patient's response to therapy and adjusting the plan as needed, ensuring that patients receive the best possible care.

With AI's ability to create highly personalized treatment plans, patients can receive more precise and effective pain management tailored to their unique circumstances.

3.5 Robotics-Assisted Pain Relief

Robotics is making a significant impact on pain management, particularly in the realm of surgery and rehabilitation. Robotic systems are enhancing precision, minimizing human error, and improving patient outcomes.

3.5.1 Robot-Assisted Surgery

In pain management, robot-assisted surgery is being used for highly precise and minimally invasive procedures, including spinal surgery, joint replacements, and nerve decompression surgeries. These robotic systems use advanced imaging and real-time data to guide surgeons, allowing for greater accuracy and reduced recovery times.

- **Benefits Of Robotic Surgery:**
  - **Increased Precision:** Robots can perform intricate procedures with a level of accuracy that minimizes the risk of complications and improves the success rate of surgeries.
  - **Minimized Incisions:** Robotic systems allow for smaller incisions, reducing tissue damage and resulting in less post-operative pain and quicker recovery times.
  - **Faster Recovery:** With enhanced precision and minimally invasive techniques, patients experience less trauma to their body, leading to faster recovery and less pain after surgery.

3.5.2 Robotic Rehabilitation Systems

Robotics is also being used in rehabilitation to help patients recover from injuries and surgeries more effectively. Robotic-assisted physical therapy devices guide patients through exercises and movements, ensuring proper technique and maximizing therapeutic outcomes.

- **Exoskeletons:** Wearable robotic devices, known as exoskeletons, are being used to assist patients with mobility issues. These devices help patients with spinal cord injuries or neurological conditions regain movement and improve their overall quality of life.

- **Robotic Therapy for Stroke And Brain Injuries:** Robotic systems are also being used to assist patients recovering from strokes or brain injuries. These systems guide patients through repetitive motion exercises, helping to rebuild motor skills and reduce pain.

Robotics is revolutionizing pain relief and rehabilitation by enhancing the effectiveness of treatments, reducing recovery time, and improving patient outcomes.

Part 2
The Physician's Perspective

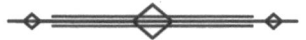

Chapter 4
Life As a Pain Specialist

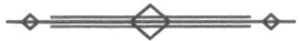

4.1 A Day in The Life Of A Pain Physician

Being a pain physician is not just a job—it's a commitment to understanding and alleviating the suffering of those who come to you seeking relief. As a pain specialist, every day is unique, shaped by the stories of patients, the complexity of their conditions, and the challenges that come with managing pain in its many forms.

My day typically begins early in the morning. Before arriving at the clinic, I spend a few minutes reviewing patient files and their progress from previous visits. It helps me get into the mindset of the day, focusing on what I can do to improve the lives of those I meet.

The first half of the day is often packed with patient consultations. These appointments are rarely predictable. Some patients are struggling with the lingering effects of surgery, others with chronic conditions like osteoarthritis or fibromyalgia, and a few with more complex neurological pain syndromes. Each of them brings a different story to the table. One might speak of pain that began after an injury years ago, while another may describe pain that seemingly appeared without warning.

Listening intently, understanding the source, and piecing together the patient's medical history helps guide me toward the most effective treatment options.

I see a lot of people dealing with pain that isn't easily visible. They may look fine on the surface, but the emotional and physical toll of living with chronic pain is often invisible. It's easy for others to misunderstand this silent suffering. That's why I prioritize taking the time to not just diagnose the condition but to truly connect with my patients. For me, it's important to make them feel heard. Pain is often as much psychological as it is physical, and understanding that balance is key.

In between patient consultations, I may consult with other specialists, particularly when patients have multiple health issues that contribute to their pain. For example, a person with chronic back pain might also suffer from hypertension or diabetes, which complicates the treatment process. It's crucial to coordinate with other experts to create a holistic treatment plan for each individual.

After lunch, I focus on reviewing new treatment options and staying updated on the latest pain management techniques. Pain medicine is a rapidly evolving field, and I make it a point to attend conferences, participate in webinars, or simply read through the latest research. Incorporating these new insights into my practice helps me provide the best care possible.

In the late afternoon, I may have follow-up appointments with patients who are undergoing ongoing treatments like injections, physical therapy, or advanced non-surgical procedures. This time is critical for assessing how well the patient is responding to treatment and making adjustments where necessary. Some patients may feel immediate relief, while others require more time or a different approach altogether.

The day ends with a reflection on everything that was discussed and learned throughout. I often find myself thinking about the people I saw and wondering how their conditions will evolve. Will the treatment plan work as expected? Will I see them again soon, or will they be able to manage their pain more independently? These are questions that stay with me, as I constantly aim to provide the best care I can.

Being a pain physician isn't easy, and the job doesn't end when the clinic doors close. The emotional weight of seeing people in pain and knowing that some won't get immediate relief can be heavy. But the moments when I can truly help someone—that's what makes every dayworth it.

4.2 Challenges In Treating Chronic Pain Patients

Chronic pain is one of the most complex and challenging areas of medicine. Unlike acute pain, which has a clear cause and usually resolves once the underlying issue is treated, chronic pain can linger for months, years, or even a lifetime. Treating chronic pain is not only about addressing the symptoms but also understanding the intricate web of factors that contribute to it. As a pain specialist, each day brings new challenges when it comes to managing this condition.

1. The Elusive Nature of Pain

One of the most significant challenges is the subjective nature of pain itself. Unlike a broken bone or an infection, where tests and scans can provide clear evidence, pain is a personal experience. It cannot be measured in the same way that physical injuries can be. When a patient describes their pain, they may use words like "sharp," "dull," "throbbing," or "burning." These descriptions are helpful but often not enough to pinpoint the exact cause.

This subjectivity makes diagnosis tricky. There is no one-size-fits-all test to confirm the presence or severity of chronic pain. Often, I rely on a detailed patient history and a combination of physical examinations, diagnostic tests, and sometimes trial-and-error treatments to uncover the root cause of the pain. Even then, there are no guarantees that the diagnosis will be 100% accurate.

2. Psychological Impact of Chronic Pain

Pain doesn't just affect the body—it also deeply impacts the mind. Chronic pain is often intertwined with psychological conditions such as depression, anxiety, and sleep disorders. Many patients experience feelings of frustration, hopelessness, and helplessness. When pain doesn't go away despite treatments, it can take a serious toll on a person's mental health.

For me, treating chronic pain means addressing both the physical and psychological aspects. This dual approach can be difficult because it requires building trust with patients, allowing them to open up about their emotional struggles. Some patients are hesitant to speak about their mental health, fearing they will be misunderstood or dismissed. As a pain physician, I strive to create a safe space for patients to share their full experiences without fear of judgment.

3. Multidimensional Causes

Chronic pain often arises from a combination of factors, including genetic predisposition, previous injuries, lifestyle choices, and environmental influences. This makes treatment even more challenging. For example, a patient with lower back pain may have developed it due to poor posture, a sedentary lifestyle, stress, and even emotional trauma. These overlapping causes complicate the treatment approach, as a single treatment modality might not address all the contributing factors.

Treating chronic pain, therefore, requires a multifaceted approach that may include medications, physical therapy, lifestyle changes, and psychological support. Even then, the journey to pain relief can be long and unpredictable. Some patients experience significant relief, while others find that their pain persists despite trying numerous interventions.

4. Managing Expectations

Another challenge in treating chronic pain patients is managing expectations. In an era where quick fixes are often promised, patients may come in expecting immediate relief. However, managing chronic pain is rarely a quick process. It often requires patience, persistence, and a willingness to try different approaches.

Educating patients about the nature of chronic pain is essential. I spend a significant amount of time explaining that while treatment can improve their quality of life, it may not completely eliminate the pain. This can be difficult for patients to accept, especially when they have been dealing with pain for many years. Helping them understand that pain management is about improving functionality and making life more manageable is crucial.

5. Finding The Right Treatment

The range of treatment options available for chronic pain is vast, but no single treatment works for everyone. Medications like analgesics and anti-inflammatory drugs are often the first line of treatment, but they come with their own set of challenges, including side effects, tolerance, and dependency issues. On top of this, the opioid crisis has led to greater scrutiny of pain management practices, particularly in how medications are prescribed.

Non-pharmacological treatments, such as physical therapy, acupuncture, or chiropractic care, may provide significant relief for some patients but may be ineffective for others. Advanced interventions, like injections or nerve blocks, can be effective but come with risks and complications. Then there are newer techniques, like stem cell therapy and regenerative medicine, which are still being studied and can be costly.

The challenge lies in finding the right combination of treatments that will work for each individual. What works for one person may not work for another, and managing these trial-and-error approaches can be frustrating for both the physician and the patient.

Treating chronic pain patients is a constant learning process. Each patient is different, and their journey to finding relief is unique. The challenges are many, but the rewards are worth it when you see a patient reclaim their life, even if it's just one small step at a time. As a pain physician, the goal isn't just to eliminate pain—it's to empower patients to live fuller, more active lives despite it.

4.3 The Emotional Toll of Dealing with Suffering

As a pain specialist, one of the less-discussed aspects of my work is the emotional toll it takes on me as a physician. While we focus on the physical aspects of pain and treatment, the emotional burden of dealing with chronic pain patients can be overwhelming at times. It's easy for those outside the medical field to think of doctors as detached, objective professionals who operate purely on clinical facts, but the reality is far more human.

1. The Weight of Suffering

Chronic pain is not just a physical condition—it is an emotional one as well. Patients living with pain often feel a profound sense of isolation, frustration, and hopelessness. The constant, unrelenting discomfort they experience can leave them emotionally drained, affecting their mental health, relationships, and overall quality of life. For many, it can feel like a never-ending battle. As a physician, I feel this burden deeply.

Each patient brings their own story, and their own emotional struggles, and as their doctor, I become an integral part of their journey. I listen to their concerns, watch them fight through their pain, and feel their anxiety over the future. As much as I try to maintain a professional distance, it's impossible not to empathize with their suffering. These emotional connections are vital for building trust, but they also leave an emotional impression on me.

2. Witnessing Frustration and Despair

One of the hardest parts of my job is seeing patients who have been through numerous treatments without success. These individuals often come to me after exhausting all other options, only to find themselves facing more disappointment. Some patients have been in chronic pain for years—decades even—and their emotional health is deeply affected. They are often worn out by the long struggle, and it's heartbreaking to witness their despair. They want to live pain-free, but the road ahead seems so uncertain.

There are days when I, too, feel helpless in the face of their suffering. The frustration is not just theirs, but mine as well. I want to provide immediate relief, but the reality of chronic pain is that sometimes even the best treatments take time to work, and sometimes we don't have a perfect solution. The weight of that helplessness can be emotionally taxing.

3. The Emotional Investment in Every Patient

Pain management is often a slow and unpredictable process. This means that, as a physician, I get to know my patients intimately—sometimes over many months, sometimes even years. I watch them go through ups and downs, feeling elated when they experience relief, only to feel defeated when the pain flares up again. This cycle can take a significant emotional toll on both the patient and the doctor.

There's an emotional investment I make in each patient's journey, and sometimes the outcomes aren't what I hope for. When treatments don't work as expected, or when I can't provide the level of relief a patient desires, it's easy to feel as though I've failed them. Even though I know the complexity of chronic pain, the emotional weight of these moments can be tough to handle.

4. The Toll On Personal Life

Caring so deeply about my patients can sometimes spill over into my personal life. There are nights when I find myself thinking about a particularly difficult case—wondering if I missed something or if there's another approach I haven't tried yet. While I'm always careful to maintain a balance, the emotional toll of the job inevitably affects me.

When I come home after a long day, I often need time to decompress and shake off the emotional weight of the day. However, there are days when that weight lingers. It's hard to disconnect completely when I carry the emotional burden of patients' suffering with me. There's a sense of responsibility that stays with me long after the clinic doors close.

5. Self-Care And Emotional Resilience

Recognizing the emotional toll this work can take is important for maintaining my well-being. If I don't take care of myself, I won't be able to care for others effectively. This means making time for activities that help me unwind—whether it's spending time with loved ones, engaging in hobbies, or simply taking quiet moments for myself. Self-care isn't just important; it's essential.

Over time, I've learned the value of emotional resilience. It's crucial to acknowledge the emotional weight of the work and to take steps to manage it. I have learned to lean on colleagues for support, engage in professional development, and ensure that I maintain a healthy work-life balance. This allows me to continue providing the best care possible for my patients without compromising my emotional health.

In the end, treating chronic pain is a deeply human endeavour, not just a clinical one. It requires empathy, compassion, and emotional resilience. The emotional toll of dealing with suffering is real, but it's also what makes the work meaningful. The moments when a patient finds relief, when they regain hope, or when they express their gratitude—those are the moments that make the emotional weight worth carrying.

4.4 Building Trust with Patients

One of the most important aspects of my role as a pain specialist is building trust with my patients. Pain is not just a physical experience—it's an emotional and psychological one too. For patients to truly benefit from treatment, they need to feel safe, heard, and understood. Trust is the foundation upon which all successful treatment plans are built, and without it, the journey to pain relief becomes much more difficult.

1. Listening And Empathizing

When a patient first walks into my clinic, their main concern is often to get relief from their pain. However, before we even discuss treatment options, I make sure to listen—listen—to what they have to say. Every patient has a unique experience with pain, and it's important for me to understand not only the physical aspects of their condition but also the emotional and psychological impacts it has on their life.

Listening deeply helps me establish a connection. It shows my patients that I'm not just a doctor ticking off symptoms from a checklist; I'm genuinely invested in their well-being. Empathy plays a huge role here—patients need to feel like they're being cared for as a whole person, not just as a case to be solved.

2. Transparency And Communication

Trust is built on open communication. I believe in being transparent with my patients about their conditions, treatment options, and potential outcomes. Pain management is rarely a straightforward process, and I always make sure my patients understand that treatments may take time to show results. Setting realistic expectations from the start is key to avoiding disappointment and frustration later on.

I also take the time to explain why I recommend certain treatments, how they work, and what side effects might occur. I make sure to answer any questions my patients may have, no matter how small they seem. This openness fosters a sense of trust and ensures that the patient feels involved in their healing process.

3. Consistency And Follow-Up

Building trust is not a one-time event—it's an ongoing process. I understand that my patients will be looking to me for guidance throughout their treatment journey, and it's important to remain consistent in both my approach and my support. Consistency creates a sense of reliability, and when patients know they can depend on me, it strengthens our relationship.

Follow-up is another crucial aspect. Regular check-ins allow me to monitor progress, address any concerns, and make adjustments to the treatment plan as needed. This continual involvement shows patients that I care about their well-being and am actively working towards their relief.

4. Respect And Empowerment

Trust thrives in an environment of respect. I treat all my patients with the utmost respect, regardless of their background, condition, or circumstances. I believe in empowering my patients to take control of their healing process. This means encouraging them to be active participants in their treatment plan, explaining the benefits of lifestyle changes, and providing education on pain management techniques they can use at home.

When patients feel respected and empowered, they are more likely to open up, share their concerns, and stick with the treatment plan. It also creates a space where patients feel comfortable discussing their fears and uncertainties—critical aspects of pain management that may otherwise remain hidden.

5. Building A Long-Term Relationship

Pain management is often a marathon, not a sprint. Many of my patients have been living with chronic pain for years, and they need someone who is committed to walking alongside them for the long haul. I view the doctor-patient relationship as a long-term partnership. Over time, we build a rapport based on mutual respect and understanding, which can make the journey much easier to navigate.

There are moments when patients come back with new concerns or frustrations, and that's when the trust we've built over time becomes especially important. They feel comfortable enough to reach out, knowing that we've worked together in the past and that I'm always here to support them in their healing journey.

In essence, trust is the bedrock of my practice. It is earned through genuine care, consistent communication, and a commitment to the patient's overall well-being. Without trust, pain management becomes a distant goal; when trust is built, healing becomes a shared journey that we embark on together.

4.5 Balancing Professional and Personal Life

As a pain specialist, my job is both fulfilling and demanding. It requires emotional investment, mental focus, and a deep commitment to my patients' well-being. However, the intense nature of this work can sometimes make it difficult to maintain a healthy work-life balance. Over the years, I have learned that managing both my professional and personal life is crucial—not just for my health but also for providing the best care for my patients.

1. The Demands of A Pain Specialist's Role

Being a pain physician is rewarding, but it is far from easy. My days are filled with seeing patients, reviewing cases, coordinating with other healthcare professionals, and keeping up with the latest research in pain management. On top of that, I am also involved in administrative tasks and managing the practical aspects of running a clinic.

The emotional toll of dealing with patients with chronic pain, as we discussed earlier, adds another layer of complexity. It's not just about diagnosing and treating; it's about being present for your patients, listening to their struggles, and providing hope. By the end of the day, I often find myself mentally exhausted.

2. Setting Boundaries

One of the first lessons I learned was the importance of setting boundaries. It's easy to get caught up in the never-ending demands of the job, especially when patients are in pain and require attention. However, without boundaries, it's easy to burn out. I had to learn how to leave work at work. I make a conscious effort to set time aside for my family, for my hobbies, and myself.

Having clear boundaries helps me maintain my energy and focus, ensuring that when I am with my patients, I am fully present, and when I am off the clock, I can recharge for the next day.

3. Prioritizing Self-Care

Self-care is often overlooked in the medical profession. Doctors are often so focused on taking care of others that they forget to take care of themselves. I've come to realize that self-care is essential—not just for my well-being but for my patients' benefit as well. If I'm not physically and mentally healthy, I won't be able to provide the best care for those who rely on me.

I make sure to incorporate activities that help me recharge—whether it's exercising, reading, or simply taking quiet moments to reflect. Meditation and mindfulness practices have also helped me manage stress and maintain mental clarity. It's about finding balance and taking care of my own body and mind so that I can continue to take care of others.

4. Making Time for Loved Ones

At the heart of my personal life are my family and friends. They are my support system, and I've learned to make time for them despite my busy schedule. Whether it's a dinner with friends, a weekend getaway with my family, or simply sitting down for a conversation at home, these moments are crucial for maintaining emotional well-being.

Being able to connect with loved ones helps me stay grounded. It provides perspective and keeps me reminded of why I do what I do. It's easy to get lost in the hustle of medicine, but family reminds me of the bigger picture—the people behind the patient charts.

5. The Importance of Flexibility

Finally, flexibility has been key to balancing both worlds. Medicine is unpredictable. There are emergencies, last-minute meetings, and unexpected patient visits. I've learned to be flexible with my time—sometimes I work late, and other times I may need to rearrange my schedule to accommodate personal commitments. Flexibility allows me to handle the challenges of my profession without sacrificing personal relationships or my health.

Balancing professional and personal life is an ongoing challenge, but it is one that I've learned to navigate with time. By setting boundaries, prioritizing self-care, and making time for those who matter most, I've been able to maintain a healthy balance. It's not always easy, but it's essential for both my own well-being and my ability to provide the best care for my patients.

Chapter 5
Social Media and Medicine

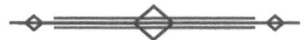

In today's digital age, social media is an undeniable force shaping nearly every aspect of life, including healthcare. It provides a platform for patients to learn, share, and connect, but it also raises serious concerns. While social media can enhance the doctor-patient relationship, it can also introduce misinformation, unrealistic expectations, and privacy issues. In this chapter, we will explore the dual role social media plays in healthcare—both as a powerful tool and a potential source of harm.

5.1 The Double-Edged Sword of Social Media In Healthcare

Social media, with its vast reach and ability to connect people across the world, has changed how healthcare professionals interact with patients. On one hand, platforms like Twitter, Facebook, Instagram, and YouTube have become valuable tools for sharing medical knowledge, offering advice, and even providing a sense of community for patients. On the other hand, these platforms are also home to countless misleading claims, pseudo-science, and non-expert advice that can harm public health.

The positive side of social media is its ability to spread accurate, evidence-based health information quickly. Doctors and medical organizations can share updates about the latest research, new treatments, and preventive measures, reaching an audience far beyond the confines of their physical practices. It also allows healthcare professionals to engage with their patients on a more personal level, offering guidance and support in ways that weren't possible in the past.

However, the dark side of social media is the ease with which misinformation can spread. Unverified health claims can go viral, causing panic or leading patients to make decisions that negatively impact their health. The lack of regulation in online spaces means anyone can post health advice, regardless of their qualifications or the validity of their claims. Healthcare providers must navigate these platforms carefully, ensuring that the information they share is accurate and balanced.

In essence, social media is a double-edged sword in healthcare: it offers both great opportunities and significant risks.

5.2 Misinformation About Pain and Its Impact

Pain management is one area where misinformation on social media is particularly harmful. Patients seeking relief for chronic pain often turn to the internet for answers, only to encounter a sea of conflicting information. They may come across claims of miracle cures or alternative therapies that promise instant results, yet these methods often lack scientific support.

Misinformation can create unrealistic expectations about the nature of pain and the treatments available. For example, some social media influencers may endorse unproven supplements or treatments, such as exotic herbs or alternative therapies, claiming they can offer fast, lasting relief from conditions like arthritis or back pain. When these treatments fail, patients may lose faith in conventional medicine and delay or avoid seeking appropriate care.

Furthermore, misinformation can lead to unnecessary self-diagnosis, where patients rely on online forums and symptom checkers rather than consulting with a healthcare provider. This can result in misdiagnosis, inappropriate treatment, and a worsening of the condition.

The spread of misinformation about pain management is not just an inconvenience—it can be dangerous. It can cause patients to ignore effective treatments in favour of unproven or harmful alternatives, delaying necessary interventions that could improve their quality of life.

5.3 The Rise of Internet Doctors and Their Influence

The advent of internet doctors—individuals claiming to provide medical advice or solutions through digital platforms—has become a significant concern. Many of these self-proclaimed experts lack proper medical training, yet they still wield considerable influence, often with large followings on platforms like Instagram,

YouTube, or Facebook. They may offer health advice, wellness tips, and even diagnose conditions based solely on online consultations.

The appeal of internet doctors is understandable. Patients looking for quick fixes or reassurance about their health may find comfort in the instant responses and easy solutions these influencers offer. However, the risks of following advice from someone without the requisite medical credentials can be serious. From recommending unverified treatments to promoting harmful products, internet doctors may mislead patients into making choices that undermine their health.

In the realm of pain management, internet doctors are particularly dangerous. Many of these online influencers promote "miracle" cures for chronic pain, claiming to offer a solution to conditions like fibromyalgia, sciatica, or osteoarthritis, often without any evidence of their effectiveness. Patients may be swayed by these promises, abandoning evidence-based treatments in favour of unproven methods.

To combat the rise of internet doctors, it is essential that healthcare professionals actively engage with the online community, sharing accurate, science-based information and establishing their credibility as trustworthy sources of health advice.

5.4 Building A Credible Online Presence as A Doctor

In the face of misinformation and the rise of internet doctors, healthcare professionals must establish a credible online presence. This means actively engaging with patients and the broader public through social media and other digital platforms while ensuring that the information shared is accurate, evidence-based, and aligned with professional standards.

Building a credible online presence begins with transparency. Healthcare providers should share their credentials, experiences, and expertise, ensuring that patients know they are engaging with a qualified professional. By openly communicating the science behind their recommendations, doctors can foster trust and combat misinformation.

Additionally, doctors can use their online platforms to provide helpful resources, such as educational videos, blog posts, and Q&A sessions. These can be tailored to the specific needs of patients, addressing common concerns, and providing scientifically supported advice. Engaging with patients in this way not only provides value but also helps establish the doctor as a thought leader in their field.

Maintaining professionalism is key. While it may be tempting to join the latest viral trends or engage in casual, off-the-cuff commentary, healthcare providers must remember that their reputation is on the line. Every post, comment, or video should reflect the same care and attention to detail that is given to in-person consultations.

Finally, healthcare professionals should actively monitor the online space for misinformation and inaccuracies. By offering counter-narratives and evidence-based information, doctors can correct myths and help steer patients toward reliable, trustworthy resources.

5.5 How Social Media Shapes Patient Expectations

Social media has fundamentally changed the way patients view healthcare. It has created a culture of instant gratification, where patients expect fast responses and immediate results. In the context of pain management, this shift in expectations can be particularly challenging.

Patients exposed to social media may have unrealistic expectations about the timeline for recovery or the effectiveness of treatments. They may come across posts or videos showing individuals who claim to have overcome chronic pain through a quick fix, whether it be an alternative therapy, supplement, or surgery. These images of immediate relief can create frustration when patients themselves don't experience similar results in the same short timeframe.

Moreover, the curated nature of social media can distort reality. Posts often showcase success stories without acknowledging the complexities of medical treatments or the effort required for long-term pain management. This can lead to disappointment when patients don't experience instant relief or find that their treatment requires more time and effort than they expected.

As healthcare professionals, it is essential to manage these expectations by educating patients about the realities of pain management. While social media can offer helpful information and support, patients need to understand that healing is often a gradual process and that long-term relief may require patience, persistence, and a holistic approach.

In this way, social media can be a tool to promote realistic expectations and empower patients with the knowledge they need to make informed decisions about their care.

Conclusion

Social media's impact on healthcare is profound, and its dual nature means it must be used with caution. On one hand, it has the power to educate, empower, and connect patients with the healthcare resources they need. On the other hand, it can perpetuate misinformation and unrealistic expectations, particularly in areas like pain management. As healthcare professionals, we must not only embrace the opportunities social media offers but also navigate its challenges by ensuring that the information we share is accurate, responsible, and accessible.

Chapter 6
The Medical Industry Ecosystem

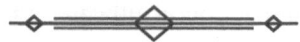

6.1 Medical Representatives: Incentives And Ethics

As a pain physician, I have often interacted with medical representatives from pharmaceutical companies. These professionals are the bridge between pharmaceutical companies and us as healthcare providers. They bring forth the latest treatments, new drugs, and even medical equipment. While their role is crucial in informing doctors about novel medical advancements, there's an underlying challenge that we must address—ethics.

Medical representatives are typically incentivized based on the products they sell. Some receive bonuses or commissions when a doctor prescribes certain medications. While I understand that this is a standard business practice, it creates a dilemma. As a doctor, my primary concern should always be the well-being of my patients, and not the sales figures of a pharmaceutical company.

Over the years, I've seen how subtle, yet persistent, pressures can arise from these relationships. It's crucial to understand that my decisions, especially in pain management, are based on evidence and the patient's unique needs, not influenced by external incentives. I ensure that the drugs or treatments I recommend are backed by solid research, and I always make my patients aware of the choices available.

Ethics in this profession are non-negotiable, and it's essential to establish clear boundaries when interacting with medical representatives. I always aim for transparency and a mutual understanding that patient welfare is paramount.

6.1.2 Navigating The Influence Of Pharmaceutical Marketing

Pharmaceutical marketing is pervasive, and as a doctor, I am continuously exposed to marketing materials, both from pharmaceutical reps and through various media channels. The challenge lies in distinguishing between informative content and promotional material designed to sell a product.

The impact of pharmaceutical marketing goes beyond the new drugs. It can shape the way doctors perceive certain treatments, sometimes swaying decisions toward those that are not necessarily the most beneficial for the patient. Over the years, I've learned to critically evaluate every marketing campaign, ad, or promotional material I come across. Just because a drug is being heavily marketed doesn't mean it is the right choice for my patient.

For example, in pain management, many pain relief medications are marketed aggressively. However, I always go back to clinical studies, patient outcomes, and evidence-based medicine to guide my treatment plans. I make it a point to filter through the noise and focus on the true needs of my patients.

As healthcare professionals, we have a responsibility to stay informed, but we also need to ensure that we are not unduly influenced by marketing campaigns that may not align with what's best for the patient.

6.1.3 The Role of Continuing Medical Education (CME)

Continuing Medical Education (CME) is a crucial part of a doctor's professional journey. It's our responsibility to stay updated with the latest treatments, techniques, and research. However, as with most things in medicine, CME programs come with their own set of challenges. A significant portion of these programs is sponsored by pharmaceutical companies, which introduces the potential for bias.

CME programs should be about educating doctors, not about promoting a specific product. Unfortunately, I've witnessed how some programs, even those that are accredited and respected, may present content in a way that favors a particular drug or device. This is a real concern, especially when it comes to pain management, where treatment options can vary widely, and patients' responses can differ significantly.

To ensure I'm providing the best care for my patients, I am very selective about the CME programs I attend. I choose those that are evidence-based and free from any bias, and I make it a point to cross-reference any new information with current clinical guidelines and peer-reviewed research.

I've also learned to be cautious about industry-sponsored CME sessions that heavily feature specific products. I always remind myself that the primary goal of CME should be to enhance patient care, not to promote sales.

6.1.4 The Changing Landscape of Healthcare Regulations

The healthcare industry is constantly evolving, and regulations around how pharmaceutical companies interact with doctors are becoming increasingly stringent. These regulations are designed to ensure that doctors prioritize their patients' welfare, rather than the interests of pharmaceutical companies. As a pain specialist, I am acutely aware of how these changes affect our practice.

Over time, regulations have placed restrictions on the kind of incentives that pharmaceutical companies can offer, the frequency of interactions between doctors and medical reps, and the transparency required in any financial relationships. These changes are vital for maintaining the integrity of the healthcare system.

It's important for all doctors, especially pain specialists, to stay up-to-date with these regulatory changes. Compliance is not just about adhering to laws but about ensuring that the care I provide is ethical and centered around my patients. These regulations help safeguard against conflicts of interest and encourage transparency, which ultimately leads to better patient outcomes.

I also make it a point to review these regulations periodically to ensure that my practice remains compliant. The landscape is always changing, and staying ahead of these changes allows me to focus on what truly matters: my patients' well-being.

6.1.5 How Doctors Can Ensure Ethical Practices

As doctors, we are the gatekeepers of healthcare, and with that responsibility comes the need for ethical decision-making. In an environment where pharmaceutical companies, medical representatives, and even patients can influence our practice, it's essential to remain grounded in our professional ethics.

For me, ensuring ethical practices means setting boundaries. I have a clear policy on how I engage with pharmaceutical representatives—any gifts, incentives, or perks are strictly avoided. I also ensure that any educational material I receive is from unbiased, credible sources, and I take the time to critically evaluate new treatment options before recommending them to my patients.

Transparency is key. I openly discuss with my patients the reasons behind my treatment choices, including the pros and cons of each option. I also disclose any potential conflicts of interest when it comes to pharmaceutical companies. By doing so, I build trust with my patients, and they understand that their health is always my primary concern.

6.2 Navigating the Grey Areas of Medical Marketing

In the modern medical landscape, marketing has become an integral part of how treatments and medications are introduced to both physicians and patients. However, the line between useful, informative marketing and potentially manipulative practices is often blurred. Navigating these grey areas of medical marketing is a challenge that every physician, especially pain specialists, must face regularly.

Medical marketing is typically aimed at educating healthcare providers and the public about new treatments, emerging technologies, and advances in pharmaceuticals. It plays a critical role in helping doctors stay updated on the latest options available to treat patients. However, the influence of marketing can sometimes stray into less transparent areas, with companies focusing on the benefits of their products while downplaying potential risks.

Pharmaceutical companies, for instance, often present clinical trials and research findings in a way that highlights the positive outcomes of their medications. While many of these findings are legitimate, it's essential to remember that marketing materials might not always include the full scope of data, especially concerning long-term side effects or potential complications. The result can be a skewed perception of what a drug can offer, which can influence how we treat our patients.

Similarly, medical device manufacturers can market their technologies with great enthusiasm, often highlighting short-term results or specific successes. Yet, when considering the implementation of a new technology in our practice, it's important to assess the full spectrum of evidence—not just the sponsored materials. This includes scrutinizing long-term safety data, comparing alternatives, and considering how well the device aligns with evidence-based practices.

One particularly tricky area is patient-focused marketing. With the rise of direct-to-consumer advertisements, patients are now more informed and, in some cases, more insistent about specific treatments they've seen advertised. This can create a dilemma for physicians, who are tasked with deciding whether a patient's request aligns with the best possible treatment for their condition. In some instances, patients may demand a particular treatment that is promoted in a way that glosses over its potential risks, putting the physician in a difficult position.

As a pain specialist, I am constantly aware of the need to protect my patients from the influence of marketing. While I believe in utilizing the latest technologies and treatments when they are genuinely beneficial, I also strive to ensure that my patients receive balanced, well-rounded information. This involves explaining not only the benefits of a treatment but also its limitations and potential risks.

Navigating these grey areas requires maintaining an ethical stance at all times. It's important to always consider the best interest of the patient, to review multiple sources of information before making treatment decisions, and to engage in ongoing professional development to ensure that we are making decisions based on the most reliable evidence available.

Ultimately, as physicians, our responsibility is to filter the noise and provide our patients with the most accurate, unbiased information. It's our duty to recognize when marketing has crossed into manipulation and to push back when a treatment or medication isn't in the patient's best interest. The ethical practice of medicine depends on our ability to separate genuine scientific advancements from the pressures of commercial interests.

6.3 Balancing Evidence-Based Medicine and Patient Demands

As a medical professional, particularly in the field of pain management, one of the most delicate aspects of treatment is balancing evidence-based medicine with the demands and desires of patients. Patients often come to us with preconceived notions about what will work for them, influenced by their personal experiences, online information, and sometimes even marketing campaigns. This creates a tension between what the scientific evidence says and what the patient expects or insists upon.

Evidence-based medicine (EBM) is the cornerstone of modern healthcare, relying on the best available research and clinical expertise to guide treatment decisions. As pain physicians, our role is to use this evidence to make informed choices about which treatments will offer the best chance of alleviating a patient's pain. However, in the real world, EBM doesn't always align with patient expectations, which can sometimes create friction.

For instance, a patient may come to the clinic asking for a specific medication or treatment they've heard about, perhaps from a friend or from an online source. They may have read testimonials of miraculous results, but the evidence behind the treatment may not be as strong as the claims suggest. It's our responsibility to navigate these expectations carefully, explaining why certain treatments may or may not be appropriate based on the evidence we have.

This situation can be further complicated when patients are demanding treatments that have not been proven to be effective or are not suited to their particular condition. For example, some patients may demand opioid prescriptions for chronic pain despite the growing evidence that long-term opioid use can lead to addiction, tolerance, and increased pain sensitivity. As a pain specialist, it is essential to balance a patient's request with the knowledge that opioids may not be the best solution for long-term pain management.

The challenge here is twofold: we must respect the autonomy of the patient while also protecting them from harm. A key part of this is effective communication. We must take the time to explain the scientific basis of treatment options and the potential risks associated with certain choices. At the same time, we need to acknowledge and address the patient's fears, frustrations, and desires. Pain is deeply personal, and our patients often turn to us as a last resort after having explored various other options.

It is also important to incorporate a holistic approach, where we look at the broader picture of a patient's health and well-being. This might mean suggesting physical therapy, psychological counselling, or lifestyle changes in addition to or instead of pharmaceuticals. Patients often appreciate the inclusion of non-invasive treatments, which not only aim to alleviate pain but also empower them to take control of their health. It's about finding that balance between respecting a patient's wishes and adhering to what the evidence tells us is most likely to lead to successful outcomes.

Moreover, there are times when patients may demand immediate results, which can be challenging. While we, as pain specialists, are committed to providing relief, we must also help patients understand that long-term pain management is often a process, not a quick fix. Our role is to guide them through this journey, offering realistic expectations while setting a course for long-term relief that may involve a combination of treatments and therapies.

Ultimately, balancing evidence-based medicine with patient demands requires a nuanced, patient-centered approach. It's about building trust, communicating effectively, and making the patient feel heard while also ensuring they understand the limitations and benefits of their treatment options. By navigating these waters carefully, we can ensure that we provide the highest standard of care while maintaining the integrity of evidence-based practice.

6.4 Surgeons Vs. Pain Physicians: Collaborations Et Conflicts

In the world of healthcare, collaboration between different specialties is essential for providing comprehensive care to patients. However, when it comes to pain management, there is often a noticeable divide between surgeons and pain physicians. Both play vital roles, but our approaches and treatment philosophies can sometimes create tension. Understanding this dynamic is crucial for fostering a collaborative and patient-centered environment.

As a pain physician, my primary goal is to alleviate suffering without resorting to invasive procedures unless absolutely necessary. Pain management is about providing long-term solutions through a combination of therapies, lifestyle changes, and, when appropriate, medications. It is a holistic approach that often seeks to avoid the operating table, focusing instead on non-surgical methods like physical therapy, interventional procedures, and behavioural therapy.

On the other hand, surgeons typically view pain through the lens of surgical intervention. They are trained to diagnose structural issues and offer surgical solutions to fix them. For conditions like herniated discs or severe joint degeneration, surgery may seem like the only viable option. Surgeons are skilled in providing immediate relief, but they may not always address the underlying causes of chronic pain, which can persist even after surgery.

However, there are many cases where surgery may not be needed, yet patients opt for it because it appears to be the only solution offered. For instance, when patients experience joint or back pain, their immediate instinct is often to think about surgical options as a "quick fix." Yet, pain management treatments without surgery can be just as, if not more, effective in many cases. Techniques like spinal injections, nerve blocks, physical therapy, and lifestyle modifications can provide lasting relief without the need for invasive surgery. As a pain physician, I have seen countless patients who, after exploring non-surgical options, are able to manage their pain successfully without undergoing surgery. This is a crucial point to understand, as not every pain issue requires an operation to resolve.

The conflict arises when a patient is referred to me for pain management after surgery, only to find that the pain persists despite the operation. In many cases, I encounter patients who have undergone surgeries that failed to address the full scope of their pain. This is where the expertise of a pain physician becomes critical. While a surgeon may focus on the mechanical or structural aspects of pain, I work to manage the multifaceted nature of chronic pain, which often involves psychological, neurological, and environmental factors.

Despite these differences, collaboration between surgeons and pain physicians is essential. I have always believed that both specialties bring unique strengths to the table, and working together can provide the patient with the best possible outcome. For instance, there are cases where surgery is necessary, but the post-operative pain management needs to be carefully coordinated to ensure that the patient's recovery is not hindered by uncontrolled pain. Surgeons and pain physicians can collaborate by creating a joint treatment plan that includes both surgical intervention and comprehensive pain management strategies.

The most effective collaborations I've seen occur when there is mutual respect between surgeons and pain specialists. Surgeons often refer patients to me when they realize that pain is not solely the result of a mechanical issue but also involves neuropathic or musculoskeletal components that require different forms of management. In return, I may refer patients to surgeons when surgical intervention is genuinely the best option. This synergy ensures that patients receive a treatment plan tailored to their specific condition.

However, the collaboration can sometimes be strained by miscommunications or misunderstandings. Surgeons may view pain physicians as being too conservative, and pain specialists may feel that surgeons take too aggressive an approach. This divide can lead to delays in treatment and dissatisfaction among patients. As pain specialists, it's crucial that we bridge this gap by being clear in our communication and always prioritize the patient's best interests.

One challenge I've encountered is when patients are caught between conflicting advice from a surgeon and a pain physician. For example, a patient who has undergone surgery may be told by their surgeon that the pain should have resolved by now and that further treatment isn't necessary. At the same time, I may identify underlying issues such as nerve damage or soft tissue injuries that could be contributing to ongoing discomfort. In these cases, it's important for me to work with the surgeon, not against them, by sharing my findings and suggesting complementary treatment strategies that could help the patient heal holistically.

Another source of conflict can be the financial incentives tied to certain treatments. Performing surgeries often earns surgeons more than providing conservative treatments or managing postoperative pain. On the other hand, pain specialists tend to have a more consistent, lower-fee structure, with payments often tied to outpatient consultations or non-invasive procedures. This economic disparity can sometimes cloud judgment and make collaboration more challenging. As a result, it's crucial to separate financial incentives from clinical decisions, ensuring that every action taken is in the patient's best interest.

In my practice, I have always made it a priority to engage with surgeons in an open and collaborative manner. I often attend multi-disciplinary meetings and discuss complex cases with my surgical colleagues. By doing so, we build a rapport and understanding that helps us navigate potential conflicts and disagreements more effectively. In the end, the success of any patient's treatment plan lies in the ability of the healthcare providers to work as a cohesive team, respecting each other's expertise while keeping the patient's well-being at the center.

Ultimately, the relationship between surgeons and pain physicians should not be one of competition but one of cooperation. We both have a role to play in the patient's journey, and when we come together, we can provide the best care possible. I always remind myself and my colleagues that no matter how different our approaches may be, our shared goal is to improve the quality of life for our patients.

The patient comes first, and by working together, we can offer them the best outcomes possible, whether that means surgery, pain management, or a combination of both.

Part 3
Empowering Patients

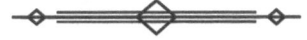

Chapter 7
Taking Charge Of Your Pain

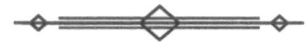

7.1 Patient Education: Understanding Your Condition

When it comes to managing pain, knowledge is power. One of the first steps in taking control of your pain is understanding the condition that's causing it. Whether you're dealing with chronic back pain, arthritis, or a complex neurological issue, learning as much as you can about your diagnosis empowers you to make informed decisions about your treatment options.

As a pain specialist, I often emphasize to my patients that understanding their condition is crucial not only for effective pain management but also for reducing feelings of anxiety or helplessness. Pain can be overwhelming, and when you don't fully understand why you're experiencing it, it can make the situation even more distressing. But when you have a clear grasp of what's happening in your body, you can approach pain management with more confidence and a sense of control.

First, it's essential to distinguish between acute and chronic pain. Acute pain is usually a temporary response to an injury or illness, signalling that something is wrong in the body. Once the underlying cause heals, the pain typically subsides. Chronic pain, on the other hand, persists for weeks, months, or even years. This type of pain is often a result of ongoing conditions like osteoarthritis, nerve damage, or fibromyalgia and may not have a clear, single cause.

Understanding the specific mechanisms behind your pain is key. For instance, if you're dealing with musculoskeletal pain, it's important to understand how muscles, ligaments, and bones work together to support your body. If you have a nerve-related condition, such as sciatica, learning about the way nerves transmit pain signals can help you better manage flare-ups. The more you know about the physical processes at play, the better equipped you are to manage your pain effectively.

Patient education also involves understanding the treatment options available to you. As a pain physician, I guide patients through various therapies, from traditional medication management to non-invasive procedures like physical therapy, and cognitive behavioural therapy. In some cases, more advanced treatments like nerve blocks or regenerative medicine may be appropriate. But knowing what each treatment entails—how it works, its potential benefits, and any associated risks—helps you make informed decisions about your care.

Additionally, understanding the impact of lifestyle factors on pain management is crucial. Nutrition, exercise, stress management, and sleep all play a significant role in how pain is perceived and managed. For instance, certain foods can have anti-inflammatory properties that may help reduce pain, while regular physical activity can strengthen muscles and improve flexibility, preventing future pain episodes. Stress, on the other hand, can exacerbate pain, so learning techniques to reduce stress, like mindfulness and meditation, can be beneficial.

Finally, it's essential to recognize that pain management is a journey. It involves trial and error, and there may be setbacks along the way. However, with the right knowledge, you can proactively, approach your pain management plan adjust it as necessary and collaborate with your healthcare team to find the most effective solutions.

Understanding your condition isn't just about learning medical terminology or understanding the latest treatments; it's about gaining a sense of agency. Pain may be a part of your life, but it doesn't define you. By educating yourself, you're taking the first step in becoming an active participant in your own healing process, which is a powerful tool for long-term relief.

7.2 How to Communicate Effectively with Your Doctor

Effective communication with your doctor is one of the most important steps you can take in managing your pain and improving your health. Many patients feel overwhelmed or unsure about how to express their symptoms, ask questions, or fully engage in their treatment plan. As a pain specialist, I've found that clear, open communication is essential to building a strong doctor-patient relationship and ensuring that you receive the best care possible.

Here are some strategies to help you communicate more effectively with your doctor:

1. Be Honest and Clear About Your Symptoms

It's crucial to be as honest and detailed as possible when describing your pain to your doctor. Pain is a highly subjective experience, and it can be difficult for a physician to assess it without accurate information. Start by describing the type of pain you're experiencing—whether it's sharp, dull, burning, aching, or throbbing. Also, mention how often it occurs, how long it lasts, and any activities or positions that make it better or worse.

Using a pain scale (from 0 to 10, where 0 is no pain and 10 is the worst pain imaginable) can also help your doctor gauge the intensity of your discomfort. For chronic pain, tracking your pain levels over time and keeping a pain diary can provide valuable insights into patterns or triggers that may not be immediately obvious.

2. Share Your Medical History and Lifestyle Factors

Your doctor needs to understand not just your current symptoms but also your medical history. Conditions such as diabetes, high blood pressure, and heart disease can all affect pain management. If you've had surgeries, injuries, or significant health events in the past, make sure you share those as well.

Equally important are lifestyle factors that can influence your pain, such as your level of physical activity, diet, sleep patterns, and mental health.

3. Ask Questions.

It's natural to have questions about your diagnosis, treatment options, and the potential side effects of medications or therapies. Don't hesitate to ask your doctor for clarification. If something is unclear, ask them to explain it in simpler terms, or ask for written information. The more you understand your condition and your treatment options, the more empowered you will feel in managing your pain.

Some important questions to consider asking your doctor might include:

- What are the underlying causes of my pain?
- Are there non-invasive treatments available to manage my condition?
- What are the potential side effects or risks of the prescribed medications or procedures?
- How long will it take to see improvement?
- Are there lifestyle changes that could help alleviate my pain?

4. Be Open About Your Treatment Preferences.

Pain management is not a one-size-fits-all approach. While some patients may prefer medication-based solutions, others may be more interested in non-surgical treatments, such as physical therapy, or cognitive behavioural therapy. Be open with your doctor about your preferences and any concerns you have about specific treatments.

In some cases, it's important to express your preferences regarding the goals of treatment. For instance, some patients might prioritize immediate relief, while others may prefer long-term solutions that address the root cause of their pain. By discussing these preferences, your doctor can help develop a treatment plan that aligns with your needs and values.

5. Follow Up and Be Proactive

Pain management often requires ongoing adjustments to your treatment plan. If something isn't working or if your pain changes, it's important to follow up with your doctor. Similarly, if you start to notice improvements or feel better, keep your doctor informed so they can adjust your treatment accordingly.

If you're undergoing make sure to stay engaged and follow your doctor's instructions closely. Attending follow-up appointments and staying consistent with prescribed therapies can significantly improve your outcomes.

6. Manage Expectations and Stay Patient

Effective communication also involves setting realistic expectations. Pain relief, particularly in cases of chronic pain, may take time. It's important to be patient with the process and understand that there may be trial and error involved in finding the most effective treatment for you. If your doctor suggests multiple options or refers you to a specialist, try to stay open-minded and trust that these steps are all part of finding the best solution for your situation.

7. Advocate For Your Needs

Finally, it's essential to be an advocate for your health. If you feel that your concerns are not being addressed or that your pain is not being taken seriously, don't be afraid to ask for a second opinion or request a referral to a specialist. Your health is your responsibility, and you deserve to have a doctor who listens to you, respects your concerns, and collaborates with you to develop a treatment plan that works for you.

Effective communication is the cornerstone of a successful doctor-patient relationship. By being clear, honest, and proactive in your conversations with your healthcare provider, you can ensure that yo recee the best possible care and take an active role in managing your pain. Whether it's discussing treatment options, setting expectations, or simply asking for clarification, your voice matters, and your doctor is there to work with you to find the best path forward in your journey toward pain relief.

7.3 Setting Realistic Goals for Pain Relief

When it comes to managing pain, especially chronic pain, one of the most important steps you can take is setting realistic goals. Many patients come into pain management with high expectations, hoping for immediate or complete relief. While it's natural to want to be pain-free, it's important to understand that pain management is often a long-term process that involves steady progress, not an instant fix. By setting realistic and achievable goals, you can better manage your expectations, stay motivated, and ultimately improve your quality of life.

As a pain specialist, I often work with my patients to help them establish clear, achievable goals that align with their specific pain conditions and lifestyle. Here's how you can set realistic goals for your pain relief journey:

1. Understand The Nature of Your Pain

Before setting goals, it's crucial to fully understand the nature of your pain. Is it acute or chronic? Is it related to a specific injury or condition, or is it a symptom of something more systemic? The more information you and your doctor have about the cause of your pain, the more effective your goals will be.

For example, if you have a condition like osteoarthritis, the focus of your goals will likely be on managing flare-ups and improving mobility. If your pain is related to muscle strain or stress, your goals may revolve around reducing muscle tension and preventing recurrence. Understanding the cause of your pain will allow you to set realistic goals that are tailored to your specific situation.

2. Set Short-Term and Long-Term Goals

Pain management is rarely a quick fix. It's important to set both short-term and long-term goals. Short-term goals will help you stay motivated and give you small wins along the way. These might include things like reducing your pain level by a specific number of points on a pain scale, improving your range of motion, or being able to complete daily activities with less discomfort.

Long-term goals, on the other hand, involve a broader vision for your overall well-being. These might include achieving a level of pain control that allows you to engage in social activities, return to work, or resume physical exercise. Long-term goals should always remain flexible because chronic pain can be unpredictable, but having a vision for the future can provide you with hope and direction.

3. Make Your Goals SMART

A great way to ensure your goals are realistic and achievable is to use the SMART criteria. SMART goals are:

- **Specific:** Clearly define what you want to achieve. Instead of saying, "I want less pain," specify how much less pain, and in what context. For example, "I want to reduce my pain level from 7/10 to 4/10 while walking."

- **Measurable:** Ensure that you can track your progress. Using a pain scale or measuring improvements in mobility can help you assess whether you're moving in the right direction.

- **Achievable:** Your goals should be challenging but realistic. Aim for progress, not perfection. If your pain level is a 9/10, it may not be realistic to set a goal of being completely pain-free within a few weeks. Instead, aim for small, gradual improvements.

- **Relevant:** Your goals should be aligned with your needs and lifestyle. If your primary concern is the inability to perform basic daily tasks, then that should be your focus rather than striving for an ambitious fitness goal in the beginning.

- **Time-bound:** Set a timeline for your goals. Having a target timeframe can help keep you accountable and motivated. For example, "I want to reduce my pain to a 5/10 level within 3 months" is a more manageable goal than setting an open-ended expectation.

4. Be Patient and Flexible.

Chronic pain can be frustrating, and progress is often slow. It's essential to be patient with yourself and recognize that healing and improvement take time. There may be setbacks along the way—flare-ups, changes in pain intensity, or new symptoms arising. These are natural parts of the journey, and they do not mean that your efforts are failing.

If you find that a goal is no longer relevant or feasible due to changes in your condition, work with your doctor to adjust it. Flexibility is key when managing chronic pain, and being open to adjusting your goals will help keep you focused on continuous improvement rather than perfection.

5. Focus On Function, Not Just Pain Relief

While pain reduction is often the primary goal, it's also important to focus on improving your function. In many cases, the goal isn't necessarily to eliminate pain, but to regain the ability to do the things that matter most to you. Whether it's playing with your children, walking a mile, cooking dinner, or working at your desk, improving your functionality can significantly improve your overall quality of life.

Your goals should incorporate not only pain reduction but also functional improvement. For example, instead of just aiming to reduce pain, you might set a goal to "be able to walk for 30 minutes without significant pain," or "be able to bend down to tie shoes without discomfort."

6. Collaborate With Your Healthcare Team

Pain management is rarely a solo endeavour. Whether you're working with a pain physician, physical therapist, psychologist, or other healthcare providers, it's essential to work together as a team. Your doctor can help you set realistic goals based on their expertise and understanding of your condition. They can also monitor your progress, adjust your treatment plan, and offer new options if necessary.

Don't be afraid to share your goals with your healthcare team. Let them know what's important to you, whether it's returning to work, engaging in hobbies, or simply reducing daily pain levels. By collaborating, you ensure that everyone involved is on the same page and working toward your best possible outcome.

7. Celebrate Small Wins

Setting and achieving realistic goals is an empowering process, and it's important to celebrate the small victories along the way. Every reduction in pain, every increase in function, and every day you feel more in control of your condition is a success. Acknowledging these small wins will keep you motivated and remind you that progress is possible, even if it feels slow at times.

Setting realistic goals for pain relief is a vital part of the journey toward managing and improving your condition. By understanding your pain, creating SMART goals, being patient and flexible, and collaborating with your healthcare team, you can take proactive steps toward a better quality of life. Remember, the journey toward pain relief is a marathon, not a sprint—take it one step at a time and celebrate every milestone along the way.

7.4 Pain Diaries: A Tool for Tracking And Managing Pain

One of the most effective yet underutilized tools in pain management is the **pain diary**. This simple yet powerful technique allows patients to actively engage in tracking their pain levels, identifying patterns, and providing essential information to healthcare providers. As a pain specialist, I often encourage my patients to maintain a pain diary, as it offers a deeper understanding of their condition and helps in devising a more personalized treatment plan.

A pain diary is essentially a log where patients record their pain experiences—when the pain occurs, its intensity, what activities or circumstances may have triggered or alleviated it, and any other relevant details. While it may seem like a minor effort, the data gathered from a pain diary can provide immense insights that significantly impact pain management strategies.

Here's how keeping a pain diary can be an invaluable tool for both patients and their healthcare providers:

1. Identifying Pain Triggers and Patterns

Chronic pain often has triggers—specific activities, environmental factors, or even emotional states—that either worsen or alleviate the pain. A pain diary helps patients recognize these patterns and understand their pain better. For example, a patient might notice that their pain worsens after prolonged sitting or after a stressful workday. By tracking such patterns, patients can make lifestyle modifications to avoid triggers or take preventive measures.

For instance, a patient with lower back pain might discover that bending down repeatedly during the day increases their pain, or they may realize that stretching or doing specific exercises helps alleviate the discomfort. Identifying these patterns early on is essential in managing pain more effectively.

2. Improving Communication with Your Healthcare Provider

A pain diary acts as a communication bridge between you and your healthcare provider. It allows you to accurately share how your pain fluctuates, how it responds to different treatments and the impact it has on your daily life. When I work with patients, I often review their pain diaries to look for trends that might not be immediately obvious in a clinical setting. It helps me understand the nuances of their pain and guide them toward the most effective treatment options.

A well-kept pain diary can also help healthcare providers identify when and how their treatments are working. For example, if a patient is undergoing physical therapy or taking medication, a pain diary can reveal whether the treatment is helping in the long term or if adjustments need to be made.

3. Understanding The Impact of Pain on Daily Life

Pain is not just a physical experience—it affects mental health, emotional well-being, and daily activities. By documenting your pain, you can track how it interferes with your ability to work, socialize, sleep, or perform other daily tasks. This information is crucial because it paints a full picture of how pain affects your life, which can help healthcare providers develop a more holistic treatment plan.

For example, a patient may note in their diary that their pain keeps them awake at night, making it difficult to concentrate at work the next day. This provides useful information that may lead to addressing sleep-related issues, pain relief before bedtime, or adjusting medications.

4. Monitoring The Effectiveness of Treatments

Keeping track of pain levels and any changes in the treatment regimen allows patients to monitor the effectiveness of their prescribed treatments. If a new medication, therapy, or lifestyle change has been introduced, the pain diary can provide immediate feedback on whether the changes are helping, worsening the pain, or having no effect at all.

A good practice is to record pain levels on a scale of 1 to 10, noting any changes, and paying attention to how long relief lasts after treatments. For instance, if a patient has been prescribed a new medication, they can document whether their pain decreases or if there are side effects like drowsiness or nausea. This information can be shared with their doctor to make any necessary adjustments.

5. Creating An Actionable Treatment Plan

With detailed insights from a pain diary, both patients and healthcare providers can create a more actionable and personalized pain management plan. Whether it involves medication, physical therapy, lifestyle changes, or mental health support, having concrete data helps guide decisions that are more likely to lead to pain relief.

For example, if a pain diary indicates that exercise relieves pain during the day but worsens at night, the healthcare provider may suggest different timing or types of exercise. Similarly, the diary might reveal that certain foods, stress, or weather conditions trigger flare-ups, guiding a nutrition plan or stress management strategy.

6. Psychological Benefits of Tracking Pain

Keeping a pain diary can also have psychological benefits. Many patients feel frustrated or overwhelmed by the constant battle with pain, and a pain diary can serve as an outlet for those emotions. It gives patients a sense of control over their pain, as they can actively document their experiences and track their progress. It can also serve as a motivational tool, as it allows patients to look back and see small improvements over time, which can be reassuring in the face of chronic pain.

7. How To Keep a Pain Diary

While a pain diary can take several forms, it's most effective when it's kept consistent and organized. Here are some tips for keeping an effective pain diary:

Daily Entries: Aim to record your pain levels and related details at least once a day, ideally at the same time every day. It's also useful to note any variations in pain throughout the day.

Pain Scale: Use a simple 1-10 pain scale to quantify pain intensity, with 1 being no pain and 10 being the worst pain imaginable. This helps create an objective measure that both you and your healthcare provider can reference.

- **Describe the Pain:** Don't just note how intense the pain is; describe its nature—whether it's sharp, dull, throbbing, or burning. These descriptors can give your doctor valuable insights into the type of pain you're experiencing.

- **Triggers and Relief:** Record any activities, foods, medications, or other factors that seem to trigger or alleviate your pain. This will help in identifying patterns.

- **Mood and Functionality:** Note how your pain affects your mood, daily activities, and quality of life. Is it affecting your sleep or causing anxiety? Does it prevent you from engaging in activities you enjoy?

8. Using Technology for Your Pain Diary

If you're tech-savvy, there are several apps available that can help you track your pain. These apps can allow for more detailed recordkeeping and offer features like reminders, progress graphs, and easy sharing with your doctor. Some popular apps even let you track medications and treatments alongside your pain logs, providing a comprehensive view of your health.

A pain diary can be one of the most useful tools in your pain management arsenal. It helps you understand your condition better, facilitates communication with your healthcare provider, and allows for more personalized and effective treatment. Whether you're managing acute pain or living with a chronic condition, keeping a pain diary offers valuable insights that can lead to better control and improved quality of life.

7.5 Red Flags That Need Urgent Medical Attention

While chronic pain can often be managed with appropriate treatment and lifestyle changes, there are certain symptoms or changes in pain patterns that may signal a more serious underlying condition. These "red flags" should never be ignored, as they may indicate the need for urgent medical attention. As a pain specialist, it's important for patients to be aware of these signs so that they can seek help promptly and avoid complications.

Below are some common red flags that may require immediate evaluation by a healthcare provider:

1. Sudden Onset of Severe Pain

If you experience sudden, sharp, or excruciating pain that is unlike your usual symptoms, it's important to take it seriously. For instance, if you suddenly feel a sharp pain in your chest, head, or abdomen or experience intense back pain, it could indicate a serious medical condition like a heart attack, stroke, or organ rupture. Immediate medical evaluation is essential to rule out life-threatening conditions.

2. Pain That Worsens Over Time

Pain that gradually intensifies, especially if it becomes progressively worse over days or weeks, can indicate an underlying issue that requires prompt medical attention. This could be a sign of an infection, tumour, or spinal cord compression. If the pain is worsening despite your treatment or self-care efforts, you should contact your healthcare provider to investigate the cause.

3. Numbness, Weakness, Or Loss of Function

Pain that is accompanied by sudden numbness, weakness, or loss of function in the limbs (arms, legs, hands, feet) should be considered an urgent concern. This could be indicative of nerve compression, a herniated disc, or a neurological condition such as a stroke. If you experience these symptoms, seek immediate medical help to prevent long-term damage or complications.

4. Loss Of Bladder or Bowel Control

If you experience a sudden inability to control your bladder or bowels, it could indicate severe spinal cord compression or cauda equina syndrome—both of which are medical emergencies. These conditions require immediate surgical intervention to prevent permanent nerve damage and loss of function.

5. Unexplained Weight Loss

Unexplained weight loss, particularly when accompanied by chronic pain, could indicate a serious health condition, such as cancer, infection, or autoimmune diseases. If you're losing weight without trying or have other symptoms like fatigue, fever, or unexplained swelling, it's important to seek medical attention for further investigation.

6. Pain With Fever or Infection

If your pain is accompanied by a fever, redness, or swelling, it may suggest an infection. Infections can cause localized pain and inflammation, and if left untreated, they can spread and become life-threatening. For instance, an infection around a joint, bone, or surgical site could lead to sepsis if not addressed promptly.

7. Difficulty Breathing or Chest Pain

Chest pain that radiates to the arm, jaw, or back, combined with difficulty breathing, dizziness, or sweating, could be indicative of a heart attack or other cardiovascular emergency. If you experience these symptoms, it is crucial to seek immediate medical attention to prevent life-threatening complications.

8. Sudden, Unexplained Headache

A sudden and severe headache, often referred to as a "thunderclap" headache, could indicate a neurological emergency, such as a brain aneurysm or stroke. It's important to seek medical attention immediately if you experience a headache of this intensity, especially if it's accompanied by vision changes, confusion, or difficulty speaking.

9. Severe Abdominal Pain

Severe abdominal pain that is sudden or worsening could be a sign of a medical emergency such as appendicitis, pancreatitis, or a perforated organ. If the pain is accompanied by nausea, vomiting, or fever, it's crucial to seek urgent medical care.

10. Swelling, Redness, Or Warmth in A Joint

If a joint becomes suddenly swollen, red, and warm, it may indicate an infection or inflammation such as septic arthritis or gout. In some cases, these conditions can lead to joint damage or systemic infection if not treated promptly. Urgent medical care is required to determine the cause and prevent complications.

11. Unusual Or Persistent Pain After an Injury

If you experience pain after an injury that persists longer than expected or worsens, it could indicate a fracture, ligament tear, or other serious injury. A thorough evaluation is necessary to ensure proper diagnosis and treatment and prevent long-term disability.

12. Pain That Spreads to Other Parts Of The Body

If your pain begins in one area but then spreads to other parts of the body (e.g., pain starting in the back and radiating down to the legs or arms), it could indicate nerve involvement or a serious condition like a herniated disc, sciatica, or even a heart attack. Early intervention is important to prevent further complications.

13. Changes In Your Pain's Pattern

If your pain, which was previously manageable or stable, suddenly changes in pattern—becoming more frequent, constant, or severe—it could be a sign that your condition has progressed or worsened. For example, if a patient with a history of chronic neck pain begins to experience pain radiating to the arm or sudden weakness, it might indicate a more serious condition requiring prompt attention.

14. Pain That Does Not Respond to Treatment

If you are receiving treatment for pain but it continues or intensifies, this is a red flag that warrants further investigation. This could indicate an error in the initial diagnosis or a need to modify the treatment plan. It's important to communicate this to your healthcare provider so they can reassess the situation and potentially order further tests.

What To Do If You Experience Red Flags

If you experience any of these red- flag symptoms, don't hesitate to seek immediate medical attention. Early intervention is crucial in preventing further complications and ensuring that your pain is treated effectively. Sometimes, urgent care may involve diagnostic tests like MRI, CT scans, blood tests, or other imaging to pinpoint the underlying cause of your pain.

It's essential to trust your body's signals and not ignore unusual or severe symptoms. While chronic pain can often be managed with appropriate treatment, sudden changes or worsening can indicate a more serious problem that requires medical attention.

Always communicate openly with your doctor about changes in your pain, and be proactive in seeking help when you feel something is wrong. Your health is your most valuable asset, and taking action early can make all the difference in managing your condition and preventing further complications.

Chapter 8
Myths And Facts About Pain

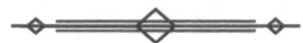

8.1 Debunking Common Myths About Pain Relief

Pain is a complex and often misunderstood phenomenon. Over time, several myths have emerged regarding pain and its relief. These myths can not only mislead patients but also prevent them from receiving the most effective treatments. As a pain specialist, it's essential to address and debunk these myths, providing patients with accurate, evidence-based information to better manage their pain.

In this chapter, we'll explore some of the most common myths about pain relief and clarify the facts to help you make informed decisions about your treatment.

1. Myth: Pain Relief Medications Always Have Serious Side Effects

While pain medications, especially opioids and strong analgesics, do carry some risk of side effects, not all pain relief options come with severe consequences. Over-the-counter (OTC) pain relievers like acetaminophen (Tylenol) and nonsteroidal anti-inflammatory drugs (NSAIDs) are generally safe when used as directed. Similarly, many non-pharmacological approaches such as physical therapy, acupuncture, or cognitive behavioural therapy (CBT) have minimal or no side effects.

The key to effective pain management is individualized care. A pain specialist will consider the benefits and risks of various treatments, tailoring a plan to the patient's needs and the type of pain they are experiencing. Not all medications or treatments carry the same risks, and proper monitoring can minimize any potential issues.

2. Myth: If You Stop Moving, Your Pain Will Improve

One of the most dangerous myths is the belief that rest is the best solution for pain, particularly when it comes to musculoskeletal pain or chronic conditions like back pain. While some initial rest may be necessary after an injury, prolonged inactivity can worsen pain by weakening muscles, stiffening joints, and reducing circulation.

Physical activity and movement are essential for pain relief and prevention. Exercise strengthens muscles, improves flexibility, and promotes endorphin production—natural substances in the body that reduce pain. A tailored exercise program, including stretches, strengthening exercises, and low-impact activities, can help alleviate pain and improve long-term outcomes. Always consult with a healthcare provider or physical therapist to ensure exercises are appropriate for your condition.

3. Myth: Surgery Is the Only Solution for Chronic Pain

Surgery is often seen as the "go-to" solution for chronic pain, especially when conservative treatments fail. However, this is a myth. Surgery is not always necessary, and in some cases, it may not even provide the desired relief. In fact, for many conditions, non-surgical treatments like physical therapy, medications, injections, and pain management interventions can be just as effective, if not more so, in relieving pain.

As a pain specialist, I frequently recommend non-surgical options first. These treatments often provide long-term relief and carry fewer risks than invasive procedures. Surgery should always be considered a last resort after other approaches have been explored.

4. Myth: Pain Is Just a Part of Aging

Many people believe that pain, particularly in the joints or back, is simply a normal part of aging. While it's true that the risk of certain conditions, such as osteoarthritis or degenerative disc disease, increases with age, this doesn't mean that pain is inevitable or that it must be accepted.

Chronic pain in older adults is often treatable. Effective pain management strategies—such as physical therapy, medication management, lifestyle modifications, and even joint injections—can significantly reduce pain and improve quality of life. Aging should not be synonymous with suffering. Seeking professional help early on can often prevent pain from becoming a permanent condition.

5. Myth: All Pain Is the Same

Not all pain is created equal. There are many different types of pain, including nociceptive pain (caused by tissue damage), neuropathic pain (caused by nerve damage), and psychogenic pain (related to emotional or psychological factors). Each type of pain has unique characteristics, and understanding the underlying cause is essential for determining the most effective treatment.

For example, nerve pain may respond better to medications like gabapentinoids or antidepressants, while inflammatory pain may benefit more from NSAIDs or corticosteroid injections. Chronic pain conditions such as fibromyalgia may require a multifaceted approach that includes medication, therapy, and lifestyle changes. Tailored treatment based on the type of pain you are experiencing is crucial for optimal relief.

6. Myth: If You Don't Feel Pain, Your Condition Is Better

Just because you don't feel pain doesn't always mean that the underlying condition has improved or healed. Pain relief doesn't always correlate directly with recovery, and many conditions (such as degenerative disc disease or arthritis) can still progress even in the absence of pain.

This myth can lead to complacency, where patients stop treatment or neglect self-care because they aren't feeling pain at the moment. It's important to continue with recommended treatments, physical activity, and lifestyle changes, even if the pain has subsided, to prevent a relapse and to support long-term healing.

7. Myth: Pain Can Always Be Completely Eliminated

While it would be ideal to eliminate all pain, especially chronic pain, the reality is that some pain may never be fully eradicated. However, this does not mean that effective management is out of reach.

The goal of pain management is often to reduce pain to a manageable level, improve function, and enhance quality of life. Many patients live with chronic pain, but with the right treatment plan, they can lead fulfilling and active lives. This may involve medications, physical therapy, lifestyle changes, and cognitive-behavioural therapy (CBT) to manage pain more effectively, even if it can't be eliminated.

8. Myth: Pain Medications Are Addictive for Everyone

While it's true that certain pain medications, particularly opioids, can be addictive, this is not the case for everyone. Many patients with chronic pain use these medications effectively without becoming addicted. The key is proper management and monitoring by a healthcare provider.

Opioids should be prescribed cautiously and only when necessary, and they should always be combined with other forms of pain management, such as physical therapy or non-opioid medications, when possible. With careful oversight and proper use, opioids can be an important part of a patient's treatment plan without leading to addiction.

9. Myth: Pain Management Is Only About Medication

Pain management is much more than simply taking medication. While medications are an essential part of pain relief for many individuals, effective pain management also involves lifestyle changes, exercise, physical therapy, mental health support, and alternative therapies like acupuncture or massage. The most successful pain management plans are comprehensive, addressing not only the physical aspects of pain but also the emotional and psychological components.

Pain management should be viewed as a holistic approach that focuses on improving the patient's overall well-being, rather than just alleviating symptoms temporarily. A well-rounded treatment plan, customized to the individual, is key to long-term success.

By debunking these myths, patients can gain a clearer understanding of pain relief and avoid unnecessary treatments or misconceptions. It's essential to approach pain management with a combination of scientific evidence, practical strategies, and open communication between patients and their healthcare providers. This knowledge empowers individuals to make informed decisions, leading to more effective treatment and better overall outcomes.

8.2 Understanding the Role Of Injections In Pain Management

Injections have become a critical part of modern pain management, offering targeted relief for various types of pain that are resistant to oral medications or physical therapy. They are often used when more conservative treatments fail, providing a way to directly address the source of pain. In this section, we will explore the role of injections in pain management, their types, benefits, and when they are appropriate.

1. Types Of Pain Injections

There are several types of injections used in pain management, each designed to address specific causes of pain. These injections deliver medications directly to the site of the pain, enhancing their effectiveness and providing faster relief.

   a. **Corticosteroid Injections:** Corticosteroids are powerful anti-inflammatory medications that can be injected into joints, tissues, or the spine to reduce inflammation and alleviate pain. They are commonly used for conditions such as arthritis, tendonitis, and herniated discs. By reducing inflammation, corticosteroid injections can provide significant relief, often lasting for several weeks to months.

   b. **Nerve Block Injections:** Nerve blocks involve injecting anesthetic or corticosteroid medications around a specific nerve or group of nerves. These injections can block pain signals from reaching the brain, providing immediate and often long-lasting relief. Nerve blocks are particularly helpful for conditions like sciatica, trigeminal neuralgia, and post-surgical pain.

c. **Epidural Steroid Injections:** Epidural injections are used to target pain in the spine. The medication is injected into the epidural space around the spinal cord and nerve roots. This is commonly used for conditions like herniated discs, spinal stenosis, and sciatica. Epidural steroid injections can reduce inflammation and pain, often providing significant relief for patients suffering from chronic back pain.

d. **Hyaluronic Acid Injections:** Hyaluronic acid injections are used primarily for joint pain, particularly in the knee. These injections aim to restore the natural lubrication in the joint, reducing friction and pain. They are often used in the treatment of osteoarthritis and can help improve mobility and function in the affected joint.

e. **Platelet-Rich Plasma (PRP) Injections:** PRP injections use the patient's blood, which is processed to concentrate platelets and growth factors. This concentrated solution is then injected into the painful area to promote healing and reduce inflammation. PRP injections are commonly used for tendon injuries, joint pain, and some types of soft tissue injuries.

f. **Botulinum Toxin Injections (Botox):** Botulinum toxin, more commonly known as Botox, can be used to treat certain types of chronic pain, such as migraines or muscle spasticity. When injected into the affected muscles, Botox can block the release of certain chemicals that contribute to pain and muscle spasms, providing relief.

2. Benefits Of Pain Injections

Pain injections offer several advantages over oral medications and other treatments. Here are some of the key benefits:

   a. **Targeted Relief:** Injections deliver medication directly to the source of pain, which means higher concentrations of the drug can be applied where it's needed most. This targeted approach ensures more effective and faster pain relief compared to oral medications that must pass through the digestive system before they can work.

   b. **Quick Onset of Action:** Injections typically provide faster relief than oral medications. For example, corticosteroid injections can reduce inflammation within hours, while nerve blocks can provide immediate pain relief by numbing the nerve directly. This rapid relief can be invaluable for patients dealing with acute or severe pain.

   c. **Reduced Systemic Side Effects:** Because the medication is injected directly at the pain site, it may reduce the likelihood of systemic side effects that are often associated with oral medications, such as gastrointestinal issues or drowsiness. This can make injections a safer and more tolerable option for some patients.

d. **Long-Lasting Relief:** Many types of injections, especially corticosteroid and hyaluronic acid injections, can provide relief for weeks or even months, reducing the need for frequent treatments. This can be particularly beneficial for patients with chronic pain conditions who have not found relief through other means.

e. **Avoiding Surgery:** In some cases, injections can provide relief from pain that might otherwise require surgery. For instance, patients with herniated discs or spinal stenosis may find significant relief through epidural steroid injections, potentially avoiding the need for spinal surgery. Similarly, joint injections can help manage arthritis pain without the need for joint replacement surgery.

3. When Are Pain Injections Appropriate?

While injections can be highly effective, they are not suitable for everyone or all types of pain. Here are some scenarios in which pain injections may be appropriate:

a. **When Conservative Treatments Fail:** Injections are often considered when other, less invasive treatments such as physical therapy, oral medications, and lifestyle modifications have failed to provide relief. If a patient's pain persists despite these efforts, injections may be used as the next step in the treatment plan.

b. **For Specific Conditions:** Injections are commonly used for conditions that involve inflammation, nerve compression, or joint degeneration, such as osteoarthritis, herniated discs, spinal stenosis, and tendonitis. They are also beneficial for chronic pain conditions like migraines, sciatica, and nerve pain.

c. **To Manage Acute Flare-Ups of Chronic Conditions:** For patients with chronic conditions like arthritis, pain injections can be helpful during acute flare-ups when pain becomes more intense and difficult to manage with regular medications. Injections can provide quick relief, allowing the patient to resume their daily activities while other treatments work to address the underlying condition.

d. **As Part of A Comprehensive Pain Management Plan:** Injections are typically not used as a standalone treatment but are integrated into a broader pain management plan. They are most effective when combined with other treatments, such as physical therapy, exercise, and lifestyle modifications. A well-rounded approach can help patients achieve long-term relief and improve their overall quality of life.

4. Risks And Considerations

Like all medical treatments, pain injections come with some risks and potential side effects. It's essential for patients to discuss these with their healthcare provider before proceeding with an injection. Some common risks include:

- **Infection:** As with any injection, there is a risk of infection at the injection site. It's crucial to maintain proper hygiene and ensure that the procedure is performed in a sterile environment.

- **Allergic Reactions:** Some patients may experience allergic reactions to the medications used in the injections. This can range from mild itching to more severe reactions, such as difficulty breathing.

- **Increased Pain:** In some cases, patients may experience temporary increased pain after the injection, which usually subsides within a few days.

- **Nerve Damage:** While rare, there is a risk of nerve damage during certain types of injections, particularly spinal or nerve block injections.

Conclusion

Pain injections can be a highly effective and valuable tool in managing chronic and acute pain. They offer targeted relief, and quick results, and may help patients avoid more invasive treatments, such as surgery. However, injections should always be used as part of a comprehensive pain management plan, in consultation with a healthcare provider, to ensure they are appropriate and safe for the patient's condition.

By understanding the role of injections in pain management, patients can make informed decisions about their treatment options, ensuring the best possible outcomes in their pain relief journey.

8.3 Can Yoga or Home Remedies Replace Medical Treatment?

When seeking pain relief, many patients are drawn to alternative approaches like yoga and home remedies. These options can provide relief, but they are not without limitations. While yoga and natural remedies offer undeniable benefits for many, they cannot always replace medical treatment, especially in severe or complex cases. **Overextending** or **misapplying** these methods could lead to complications or further injury. Here's a deeper look at their roles:

1. Yoga: A Useful Complement, But Not a Cure-All

Yoga has proven benefits for certain types of pain, including chronic back pain, arthritis, and stress-induced discomfort. However, when practiced incorrectly or excessively, it can also cause harm. People who push their bodies beyond their limits might end up with more injuries than relief. For instance, **overstretching** or improper alignment in yoga poses can strain the ligaments, tendons, and muscles, sometimes leading to serious injuries such as **ACL or PCL tears**, especially in individuals who already have pre-existing joint issues.

- a. **The Benefits of Yoga:**
    - **Increased Flexibility and Strength:** When done correctly, yoga helps to strengthen muscles and increase flexibility, which can reduce tension and alleviate pain.

- **Stress Reduction:** Yoga's emphasis on mindfulness and deep breathing can have a profound impact on reducing stress and improving the body's response to pain.

b. **Potential Risks:**
- **Misalignment And Injury:** Without proper guidance, patients may inadvertently cause more harm. For instance, certain postures, especially if done with improper technique, can exacerbate existing pain or lead to new injuries.
- **Excessive Practice:** It's tempting for some to push through discomfort, but doing so can lead to muscle strains, ligament tears, or even exacerbate joint issues.

Takeaway: Yoga can help, but it should never be used as a substitute for medical intervention when dealing with acute pain or serious conditions. Always seek proper instruction and listen to your body.

2. Home Remedies: Helpful, But Limited

Home remedies like herbal teas, heat or ice packs, and essential oils offer comfort for minor, temporary pain relief, but they are **not substitutes for medical treatment** in serious conditions. For example, while an ice pack can relieve a mild muscle strain, it won't help with the underlying cause of chronic pain such as nerve damage, arthritis, or herniated discs. Moreover, over-reliance on these remedies may delay diagnosis and treatment, allowing conditions to worsen.

a. **The Benefits of Home Remedies:**
   - **Accessibility And Cost-Effective:** Many home remedies are easy to access and inexpensive. For mild pain relief, these can be effective as complementary solutions.
   - **Natural Anti-Inflammatory Options:** Herbs like turmeric or ginger, known for their anti-inflammatory properties, can offer some relief, but only to a limited extent.

b. **The Risks:**
   - **Inadequate For Serious Pain:** Home remedies rarely address the root causes of severe or chronic pain. They might mask symptoms temporarily, but they don't treat underlying conditions that require medical intervention.
   - **Delaying Professional Care:** If patients use home remedies in place of seeking medical help, they may miss the opportunity for an early diagnosis, allowing the condition to worsen and become harder to treat.

Takeaway: Home remedies can support pain management but should never replace professional treatment. They are best used in conjunction with medical care, particularly when pain becomes chronic or more severe.

3. Finding The Right Balance

It's important to remember that yoga and home remedies can serve as **valuable tools in managing pain**, but they are most effective when used in **combination with**

medical treatments, not as replacements. For instance, if you're recovering from an injury, yoga might help with gentle stretching and improve flexibility, but it shouldn't be used in place of physical therapy or other prescribed treatments. Similarly, home remedies can offer temporary relief, but they are not sufficient for treating serious conditions like nerve damage or spinal disorders.

Conclusion:

While yoga and home remedies are beneficial as complementary treatments, **they should never replace medical intervention**, especially when dealing with serious or chronic pain. Patients should seek professional advice before pursuing these alternatives, particularly when they feel the need to stretch the limits of what is comfortable in yoga or rely too heavily on self-administered remedies. The goal is always to **balance** natural methods with medical expertise to achieve the best possible outcomes. Always remember: **listen to your body, but also trust your doctor.**

8.4 The Truth About Supplements and Alternative Medicine

In recent years, the popularity of supplements and alternative medicine has surged, offering promises of fast pain relief, enhanced health, and a better quality of life. From herbal remedies to vitamin supplements, the market is flooded with products that claim to heal a range of ailments, including chronic pain. However, the question remains: **How reliable are these treatments, and do they work?**

As a pain physician, I often encounter patients who have tried countless supplements or alternative therapies in search of relief. While some may find temporary benefits, others are left disappointed, or worse, their conditions worsen. It's crucial to understand that **not all supplements or alternative treatments are created equal**, and relying on unproven remedies can do more harm than good.

1. The Rise of Supplements In Pain Management

Supplements are a popular choice for people looking for natural alternatives to manage pain, and in some cases, they may provide certain benefits. The key word here is **certain**. There are scientifically backed supplements such as **turmeric, omega-3 fatty acids**, and **glucosamine** that have shown promise in reducing inflammation and supporting joint health. However, these benefits can vary from person to person, and their effects are not guaranteed.

   a. **Evidence-Based Supplements:**
- **Turmeric (Curcumin):** Known for its anti-inflammatory properties, turmeric has been studied for its effectiveness in managing pain, particularly in conditions like osteoarthritis. Some clinical trials show that turmeric extract can reduce pain and improve joint function, though the results are often moderate.
  - **Omega-3 Fatty Acids:** Found in fish oil, omega-3s are linked to reduced inflammation and have shown promise in managing chronic pain conditions like rheumatoid

arthritis. The evidence here is robust, but the effectiveness can depend on the individual's response.

- **Glucosamine And Chondroitin:** These are commonly used for joint pain and are believed to help with cartilage repair. While some studies suggest they may provide mild pain relief for osteoarthritis, others have found little to no effect.

However, it's essential to consult a healthcare provider before starting any supplement regimen, especially if you are already undergoing treatment for an existing condition.

b. The Dark Side of The Supplement Industry:

The supplement industry is largely unregulated, and many products available on the market have little to no scientific evidence backing their claims. You might see supplements marketed as "all-natural" or "clinically proven," but without rigorous clinical trials and scientific research, these claims are often unsubstantiated. For example:

- **Unproven Supplements:** Many herbal remedies, such as **Krill oil**, **Ginseng**, or **Devil's Claw**, are often advertised as miracle solutions for pain, but scientific evidence on their efficacy is limited or inconclusive. In some cases, these supplements may even interact with prescription medications, leading to harmful side effects.

- **Lack Of Standardization:** Unlike pharmaceuticals, supplements are not subject to the same rigorous standards for quality, purity, and potency. Some products may contain fillers, contaminants, or incorrect dosages that can be dangerous to health.

2. Alternative Medicine: Proceed with Caution

Alongside supplements, many people turn to alternative medicine practices like acupuncture, chiropractic care, and massage therapy, hoping to find relief from chronic pain. While some of these treatments are backed by anecdotal evidence and may offer **temporary relief**, they are not always effective for everyone and, in some cases, can be risky.

Acupuncture and massage are both popular alternatives for pain management, and some studies suggest that acupuncture, in particular, may help with conditions like lower back pain and osteoarthritis. However, the effectiveness of these treatments is still up for debate. Not every patient will respond to these therapies, and they should be used as complementary treatments rather than primary solutions.

a. **Chiropractic Care:** Chiropractic adjustments can help with musculoskeletal pain, especially neck and back pain. However, for some people, particularly those with certain underlying conditions, chiropractic care can lead to complications. Again, it's important to consult a medical professional before undergoing alternative treatments.

3. Understanding The Role of Evidence-Based Medicine

The bottom line with supplements and alternative medicine is that **scientific evidence matters**. While there are some well-documented and effective treatments, there is no one-size-fits-all solution for pain relief. Relying solely on alternative therapies without evidence of their effectiveness can result in patients missing out on proven, medically supported treatments.

a. How To Make Informed Decisions:

- **Consult Your Physician**: Before taking any supplement or starting an alternative treatment, speak with your doctor. They can guide you based on your specific health needs and help you make an informed decision about whether a particular treatment will benefit you.

- **Look For Evidence:** When considering any supplement or alternative therapy, look for clinical studies, trials, or research backing its effectiveness. Reliable sources like the **National Institutes of Health (NIH)** or **PubMed** provide research-backed information that can help you evaluate the claims.

- **Don't Substitute for Proven Treatments:** While supplements and alternative medicine can be a part of a broader treatment plan, they should never replace proven medical treatments, especially for serious conditions like arthritis, nerve damage, or autoimmune disorders. Pain management requires a balanced approach, combining effective medical treatments with complementary therapies where appropriate.

4. A Call for Transparency And Accountability

The world of supplements and alternative medicine is vast and often overwhelming, and the lack of regulation creates opportunities for misinformation and exploitation. As patients, we must advocate for transparency, accountability, and ethical marketing practices in the healthcare industry. As a pain physician, I stress the importance of relying on **evidence-based** treatments, and I encourage patients to question treatments that lack scientific validation.

Conclusion:

While supplements and alternative medicine can play a supportive role in pain management, they should not replace professional medical care. The most important step in finding effective pain relief is **education**—becoming an informed patient who understands the **science behind the treatments** they are considering. Look for products with **proven effectiveness**, consult with your healthcare provider, and be cautious of quick fixes that may do more harm than good. Above all, remember that your health is your responsibility, and making informed, evidence-based choices is the best way to ensure long-term relief and well-being.

Part 4
A Holistic Approach to Pain Relief

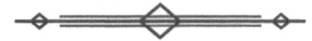

Chapter 9
The Role of Mind-Body Connection

9.1 How Stress Amplifies Pain

The connection between the mind and body is powerful, influencing our overall health in ways we may not fully comprehend. While we often focus on physical symptoms when dealing with pain, we cannot ignore the profound impact that emotional and psychological stress has on our pain experience. Stress, whether acute or chronic, can play a pivotal role in amplifying pain and making it harder to manage, often complicating the healing process.

Understanding how stress affects pain is essential in creating a comprehensive, holistic approach to pain relief. This chapter will explore the physiological mechanisms that link stress to pain and provide practical strategies for managing stress to alleviate pain.

1. The Physiological Link Between Stress and Pain

Stress triggers a series of physical and emotional responses that affect how we perceive pain. When the body is stressed, the **sympathetic nervous system**, also known as the "fight or flight" system, becomes activated.

This response is helpful in dangerous situations, preparing the body to react quickly. However, when stress is constant, as in the case of chronic stress, this system remains overactive, leading to a cascade of physical changes that can increase pain sensitivity.

- a. **The Role of Cortisol:** When we experience stress, our body releases a hormone called **cortisol**, which plays a key role in managing stress by preparing the body for action. However, prolonged exposure to high levels of cortisol can lead to a number of negative effects, including:

    - **Increased Inflammation:** Chronic stress increases the levels of inflammation in the body, which can exacerbate conditions such as **arthritis**, **back pain**, or **muscle pain**. Inflammation is a primary contributor to pain, and its persistence can make pain more intense and harder to control.

    - **Sensitization Of Pain Pathways:** Chronic stress can affect the brain's pain pathways, making them more sensitive. This means that your brain may perceive pain as being more intense or more widespread than it actually is. Over time, this process can lead to **central sensitization**, a condition where even non-painful stimuli are perceived as painful.

- b. **Muscle Tension and Stress:** Stress also causes muscle tension, particularly in areas such as the shoulders, neck, and back. When muscles are tense for long periods, it can result in **muscle**

stiffness and **muscle spasms**, which are often a direct cause of pain. This is commonly seen in people who have **chronic neck or back pain**, where stress leads to a persistent cycle of pain and tension.

2. Psychological Impact:

Stress also has significant psychological effects that contribute to the perception of pain. It can create a vicious cycle: stress causes pain, and pain causes stress. When people experience ongoing pain, it often leads to **anxiety**, **depression**, and **frustration**. These emotional responses can heighten the body's sensitivity to pain, creating a situation where emotional stress and physical pain are inextricably linked.

   a. **Anxiety And Pain:** People with anxiety disorders often experience heightened sensitivity to pain. Studies have shown that anxiety can increase the intensity of both **chronic pain** and **acute pain** episodes. This may be because anxiety triggers a state of hypervigilance, where a person is constantly on edge, interpreting normal body sensations as painful or threatening. As a result, individuals may become more aware of pain and have a lower pain threshold.

   b. **Depression And Pain:** Depression, often associated with chronic pain conditions, can contribute to a **negative feedback loop** where pain worsens depression, and depression worsens pain. Depressed individuals may experience **disrupted sleep, fatigue,** and a reduced ability to engage in activities, all of which can make pain more intense and persistent. Moreover, the lack of motivation to seek treatment or engage in pain-relief strategies may further intensify the pain experience.

3. How Stress Affects Specific Pain Conditions

Certain pain conditions are more strongly influenced by stress. Here are some examples of how stress exacerbates specific pain conditions:

- **Fibromyalgia:** Fibromyalgia is a chronic pain condition marked by widespread muscle pain, fatigue, and sleep disturbances. Stress has been identified as a major trigger for flare-ups of fibromyalgia symptoms. High levels of stress can amplify the body's sensitivity to pain, making the pain felt by fibromyalgia patients more intense.

- **Chronic Headaches and Migraines:** Stress is one of the most common triggers for headaches and migraines. Emotional and psychological stress can lead to tension headaches, while more severe stress can trigger a migraine attack. The **cortisol** released during stressful events can affect the blood vessels in the brain, leading to headache pain.

- **Back And Neck Pain:** As mentioned, chronic stress causes muscle tension, which is a major contributor to back and neck pain. Prolonged muscle tension can lead to **muscle spasms** and

muscle strain, which, in turn, can create or worsen pain in the back and neck regions.

- **Arthritis:** Stress can worsen symptoms of **rheumatoid arthritis** and **osteoarthritis**. Chronic stress leads to increased inflammation in the body, which can make joint pain, stiffness, and swelling worse.

4. Practical Strategies for Managing Stress To Alleviate Pain

Given the powerful link between stress and pain, addressing stress management is a critical part of any pain relief strategy. Here are some **effective approaches** to managing stress that can help reduce pain:

a. **Mindfulness And Meditation:** Mindfulness practices, such as meditation, have been shown to significantly reduce stress and improve pain management. Mindfulness helps individuals focus on the present moment, reducing worry and anxiety. Techniques such as deep breathing, body scans, and visualization can calm the nervous system and reduce pain sensitivity.

- **Mindfulness-Based Stress Reduction (MBSR):** This is an evidence-based program that teaches mindfulness meditation to help reduce stress. Studies have shown that MBSR can be effective in reducing chronic pain and improving emotional well-being.

b. **Cognitive Behavioural Therapy (CBT):** CBT is a form of talk therapy that helps individuals change negative thought patterns that contribute to stress and pain. By focusing on identifying and changing unhelpful thoughts and behaviours, CBT can help patients cope better with pain and reduce the emotional toll that stress takes on their body.

c. **Physical Activity and Exercise:** Exercise is a powerful stress reliever that can also help with pain management. Regular physical activity can reduce muscle tension, release endorphins (the body's natural painkillers), and improve overall mood. It also helps improve sleep quality, which is often disrupted by stress and pain.

d. **Social Support:** Social connections play a vital role in stress reduction. Having a support system of family, friends, or pain support groups can help patients manage both the emotional and physical aspects of pain. Talking with others who understand your pain can reduce feelings of isolation and help you feel more in control.

e. **Relaxation Techniques:** Techniques such as **progressive muscle relaxation**, **deep breathing exercises**, and **guided imagery** can help calm the body and mind. These techniques promote relaxation and reduce the physiological effects of stress, helping to relieve tension in the body and manage pain.

Conclusion:

The relationship between stress and pain is complex, but one thing is clear: stress has a significant role in amplifying pain, and addressing this mind-body connection is crucial for effective pain management. By understanding the physiological and psychological mechanisms that link stress to pain, patients can take proactive steps to manage stress and alleviate pain. A holistic approach to pain relief, which includes managing stress through mindfulness, exercise, therapy, and social support, can provide meaningful relief and improve the overall quality of life.

By focusing on both the **mental and physical aspects** of pain, patients can begin to break the cycle of stress and pain, leading to a more manageable and fulfilling life.

9.2 Rewiring the Brain For Pain Tolerance

The brain plays a central role in how we perceive and experience pain. While pain begins as a physical signal sent to the brain, the brain processes it and influences how it is perceived. For those suffering from chronic pain, the brain can become "wired" to interpret signals from the body as more painful or intense than they actually are. This phenomenon is often referred to as **central sensitization**, where the brain amplifies pain signals. The good news is that the brain is not set in its ways—it has remarkable **neuroplasticity**, meaning it can be rewired and retrained to better handle pain.

In this chapter, we'll explore how the brain processes pain, how chronic pain can alter the brain's response, and practical methods to **retrain the brain** to improve pain tolerance and alleviate suffering.

1. Understanding Neuroplasticity and Pain

Neuroplasticity is the brain's ability to reorganize itself by forming new neural connections. While this process is commonly associated with learning and memory, it also plays a crucial role in how the brain processes pain. When we experience pain repeatedly, the brain's pain pathways can become overly sensitized, and pain can feel much more intense or widespread than it should. This is often seen in conditions like **fibromyalgia, chronic lower back pain**, and **migraines**, where the pain persists long after the injury or inflammation has healed.

Over time, the brain learns to associate certain sensations with pain, even in the absence of an injury. This means that the brain can misinterpret normal bodily sensations (such as touch or movement) as painful. The key to breaking this cycle is understanding that the brain can be retrained to reduce its sensitivity to pain signals.

2. How The Brain Processes Pain: The Pain Pathway

To understand how the brain can "retrain" itself, we must first explore how pain is processed:

a. **Pain Reception:** When the body experiences an injury or potential harm, sensory receptors (called nociceptors) send signals to the spinal cord, which then transmits these signals to the brain. This is how the body first detects pain.

b. **Pain Modulation:** The brain has areas that can modulate or adjust the intensity of pain signals. In a healthy system, the brain can prioritize pain based on severity. However, in the case of chronic pain, this modulation system may become impaired, leading to a constant amplification of pain signals.

c. **Chronic Pain and Sensitization:** Repeated exposure to pain causes the brain's neural circuits to become more sensitive to pain signals. This heightened sensitivity is known as **central sensitization**. It means the brain becomes hyperactive and overreacts to pain stimuli, even those that would not have caused significant pain initially.

3. Rewiring The Brain for Pain Relief

Just as the brain can become sensitive to pain, it can also be trained to desensitize and tolerate it more effectively. This process of "rewiring" the brain is possible through several approaches:

a. **Mindfulness And Meditation:** Mindfulness-based practices focus on increasing awareness of the present moment without judgment. Studies have shown that mindfulness meditation can help **reduce pain perception** by calming the nervous system and altering brain activity. Mindfulness meditation activates areas of the brain involved in **pain regulation**, such as the **prefrontal cortex**, and helps reduce the brain's response to pain stimuli.

- **Example:** The practice of mindfulness meditation has been shown to activate the **anterior cingulate cortex**, a part of the brain that plays a role in emotional regulation and pain perception. Over time, regular practice can help individuals better manage chronic pain by teaching the brain not to react with heightened pain sensitivity.

b. **Cognitive Behavioural Therapy (CBT):** CBT is a widely used psychological treatment that focuses on changing thought patterns. In the context of chronic pain, CBT can help individuals recognize and modify the negative thoughts and behaviours that reinforce pain. By changing these thought patterns, the brain's emotional response to pain can be shifted, thus reducing the perception of pain.

c. **Graded Exposure and Desensitization:** Graded exposure is a technique used in physical therapy where individuals gradually and systematically expose themselves to activities or movements that may trigger pain. Over time, as the body adapts to these movements, the brain learns that they are not harmful, leading to reduced pain sensitivity.

- **Example:** If a person experiences chronic knee pain, they might start with simple leg movements or light stretching. Slowly, over time, they can increase the intensity of these movements, allowing the brain to become less sensitive to the sensation and improving pain tolerance.

d. **Virtual Reality Therapy:** Emerging research shows that **virtual reality (VR)** can be a powerful tool for managing chronic pain. By immersing patients in virtual environments, the brain can become distracted from pain signals. Virtual reality has also been shown to alter the brain's pain processing centers, effectively rewiring the brain's response to pain.

e. **Physical Therapy and Exercise:** Regular physical activity plays a vital role in managing chronic pain by releasing **endorphins** (natural painkillers produced by the body) and enhancing the brain's ability to tolerate discomfort. Through exercise, the brain can also learn that movement does not necessarily lead to pain, helping to break the cycle of fear and pain avoidance.

f. **Neurofeedback:** Neurofeedback is a technique that involves training individuals to control brain activity. It has been used to treat conditions like chronic pain by teaching the brain to reduce the intensity of pain signals. The process involves monitoring brain waves and providing real-time feedback to the individual, helping them learn how to adjust their brain activity to promote pain relief.

4. The Power of Belief and The Plato Effect

An often overlooked aspect of pain management is the role of **belief** in how pain is perceived. Research into the **placebo effect**—where patients experience real pain relief after receiving a treatment they believe will help, even if it has no therapeutic value—demonstrates the power of the mind in managing pain.

Belief in a treatment's effectiveness can activate areas of the brain associated with pain relief. For example, the brain's **opioid system**, which releases natural pain-relieving chemicals, can be activated by a person's belief in a treatment's success. This means that the mind's ability to perceive pain is not only a physical response but also a psychological one.

5. Practical Steps to Rewire The Brain For Pain Tolerance

There are several practical strategies that individuals can implement to help rewire the brain for better pain tolerance:

- **Mindfulness Meditation:** Practice daily for at least 10–20 minutes to help regulate pain perception and reduce stress.

- **Cognitive Behavioural Therapy (CBT):** Engage in therapy with a trained professional who can guide you in identifying and changing negative thought patterns related to pain.

- **Gradual Exposure:** Start with low-level activities or movements that trigger pain and gradually increase intensity, helping the brain adapt to pain triggers.

- **Physical Activity:** Incorporate regular, moderate exercise into your routine. Activities like walking, swimming, or yoga are great for building strength and tolerance to pain.
- **Positive Visualization:** Engage in guided imagery exercises where you visualize your body healing and becoming more resilient to pain.
- **Biofeedback And Neurofeedback:** Consider working with a therapist trained in biofeedback or neurofeedback techniques to help control brain activity and pain sensitivity.

Conclusion

Rewiring the brain for pain tolerance is a process that requires time, patience, and consistent effort. Through techniques like mindfulness, physical therapy, cognitive behavioural therapy, and exercise, patients can reprogram their pain responses and significantly reduce their discomfort. By recognizing the power of the mind-body connection, individuals can break free from the cycle of chronic pain and build greater resilience and tolerance to discomfort.

In the end, pain tolerance is not just about enduring the pain but learning how to change the brain's response to it, empowering individuals to regain control of their lives and well-being.

Chapter 10
Lifestyle As Medicine

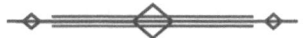

10.1 Nutrition's Role in Pain Management

Nutrition plays a critical role in managing pain, particularly chronic pain. The foods we eat can either help reduce inflammation and pain or exacerbate it. While medications and treatments are essential components of pain management, many individuals overlook the impact of diet on their overall health, including how they experience and manage pain. **Proper nutrition** not only nourishes the body but also provides essential nutrients that support recovery and reduce inflammation, two critical factors in pain management.

In this chapter, we will explore how specific nutrients, dietary patterns, and eating habits can influence pain levels, as well as practical strategies to incorporate pain-relieving foods into daily life.

1. Inflammation And Pain: The Connection

Many chronic pain conditions, such as arthritis, back pain, and fibromyalgia, are characterized by **inflammation** in the body. Inflammation occurs when the immune system responds to injury or illness, often causing pain, redness, and swelling in the affected area. While short-term inflammation is a natural healing response, **chronic**

inflammation can lead to prolonged pain and tissue damage.

Certain foods can either **reduce** or **increase** inflammation in the body. A diet rich in anti-inflammatory foods can lower inflammation, alleviate pain, and support overall health. Conversely, a diet high in pro-inflammatory foods can contribute to pain, exacerbate existing conditions, and slow down the healing process.

2. Anti-Inflammatory Foods

Several foods have been shown to possess **anti-inflammatory properties**, which can help reduce pain. These foods are rich in antioxidants, healthy fats, and essential vitamins and minerals that combat inflammation and support immune function. Some key anti-inflammatory foods include:

- **Fatty Fish (Salmon, Mackerel, Sardines):** These fish are high in **omega-3 fatty acids**, which are known to reduce inflammation and pain. Omega-3s help balance the inflammatory processes in the body and support joint health.

- **Leafy Greens (Spinach, Kale, Swiss Chard):** Rich in vitamins, antioxidants, and minerals, these greens contain compounds like **vitamin K** and **flavonoids**, which help reduce inflammation and protect cells from damage.

- **Berries (Blueberries, Strawberries, Raspberries):** Berries are packed with antioxidants like **anthocyanins**, which have been shown to reduce oxidative stress and inflammation. They also help fight free radicals in the body, promoting overall healing and pain relief.

- **Turmeric:** The active compound in turmeric, **curcumin**, has powerful anti-inflammatory and antioxidant properties. It can help reduce inflammation in the joints and may alleviate pain in conditions like arthritis.

- **Olive Oil:** Rich in **monounsaturated fats** and antioxidants, olive oil contains oleocanthal, a compound with anti-inflammatory effects that can help reduce pain, particularly in joint conditions.

- **Ginger:** Known for its anti-inflammatory properties, ginger contains **gingerols** that help reduce pain and swelling. It can be effective in managing symptoms of osteoarthritis, rheumatoid arthritis, and other inflammatory conditions.

- **Nuts And Seeds (Almonds, Walnuts, Flaxseeds):** These contain healthy fats and antioxidants that help decrease inflammation and promote heart health. Walnuts, in particular, are rich in omega-3 fatty acids.

3. The Role of Vitamin D And Calcium

Vitamin D and **Calcium** are essential for maintaining healthy bones and muscles. **Vitamin D** helps the body absorb calcium, which is crucial for bone density and strength. Low levels of vitamin D are often linked to increased pain sensitivity and musculoskeletal pain, including in conditions like **osteoporosis** and **fibromyalgia**.

Foods rich in **vitamin D** include fortified dairy products, eggs, and fatty fishlike salmon. **Calcium-rich foods**, such as dairy products, leafy greens, tofu, and fortified plant-based milks, also play an important role in preventing bone-related pain and improving overall bone health.

4. The Impact of Sugar and Processed Foods On Pain

While certain foods can help manage pain, others can worsen it. **Added sugars**, **refined carbohydrates**, and **processed foods** have been linked to increased levels of inflammation in the body. These foods promote the production of **cytokines**, which are proteins that can lead to inflammation. Chronic consumption of sugar and processed foods can worsen pain in conditions like **arthritis**, **diabetes**, and **obesity**.

Reducing or eliminating sugary and highly processed foods from your diet can help control inflammation and pain. Instead of sugary snacks, it's better to opt for **whole foods** that provide natural nutrients and antioxidants that support the body's natural healing processes.

5. The Role of Hydration In Pain Relief

Staying properly hydrated is essential for maintaining joint lubrication and reducing pain. **Dehydration** can exacerbate conditions like back pain and joint pain, as the discs in the spine rely on water to cushion and support the body's structure. Similarly, lack of hydration can affect joint fluidity, making movement painful and stiff.

Drinking plenty of water throughout the day helps maintain joint health, flush out toxins, and support the body's natural anti-inflammatory processes. In addition to water, herbal teas, and **electrolyte-rich beverages** can also promote hydration.

6. Eliminating Trigger Foods

In addition to incorporating anti-inflammatory foods, it's also important to avoid foods that may trigger inflammation and pain. Some common trigger foods include:

- **Nightshades (Tomatoes, Potatoes, Peppers, Eggplant):** These foods contain solanine, a compound that can aggravate symptoms in individuals with arthritis or joint pain.

- **Processed Meats (Sausages, Hot Dogs, Bacon):** These foods contain preservatives and chemicals that can promote inflammation and exacerbate pain.

- **Dairy Products (For Some Individuals):** While dairy can be an excellent source of calcium, some individuals with lactose intolerance or sensitivity may experience pain and inflammation after consuming dairy.

By identifying and eliminating **trigger foods** from your diet, you can help reduce chronic inflammation and improve your overall pain management.

Conclusion

Nutrition is a key component of pain management, and incorporating anti-inflammatory foods into your diet can have a profound impact on reducing pain and improving overall health. By choosing whole, nutrient-dense foods and avoiding inflammatory triggers, individuals can better manage chronic pain conditions and enhance their overall quality of life.

A balanced, well-planned diet not only provides the necessary building blocks for recovery but also supports the body's natural healing processes, helping individuals live more comfortably and actively. The power of nutrition in pain management is undeniable, and with the right choices, patients can take an active role in their pain relief journey.

10.2 Ergonomics: How to Create A Pain-Free Workspace

As a pain physician, I've seen firsthand how poor workplace ergonomics can lead to chronic discomfort and musculoskeletal issues. Many of my patients experience recurring pain in their back, neck, shoulders, and wrists, often stemming from improper desk setups and prolonged hours of sitting. In fact, workplace ergonomics plays a crucial role in either exacerbating or alleviating pain, especially in those who spend long hours in front of screens.

Ergonomics is the science of designing workspaces, tools, and tasks in a way that minimizes physical stress on the body. Creating an ergonomically sound workspace can significantly reduce the risk of developing pain or injury, leading to more comfort and productivity. Here, I'll share some essential tips for setting up a workspace that promotes optimal posture and minimizes strain on the body.

1. Understanding The Importance Of Ergonomics

For those of us working at desks for extended periods, the risk of developing musculoskeletal pain is high. Poor posture, like slouching or leaning forward while using a computer, can lead to pain and discomfort. Over time, these bad habits can cause serious injuries, including chronic back pain, carpal tunnel syndrome, and even eye strain.

From an evidence-based perspective, creating an ergonomic workspace is one of the most effective ways to prevent such conditions. Not only does it help reduce physical discomfort, but it can also improve focus and productivity. When you're not distracted by aches and pains, you can work more efficiently and feel better throughout the day.

2. Proper Chair Setup

A **good chair** is the cornerstone of a pain-free workspace. In my practice, I emphasize the importance of maintaining the natural alignment of the body, especially the spine, while sitting. If the chair doesn't provide proper support, it can lead to strain and discomfort in the lower back, neck, and hips.

Here are a few essential factors to consider when setting up your chair:

- **Seat Height:** Your feet should be flat on the floor, and your knees should be at a 90-degree angle. If your chair is too high or low, it can cause strain on your legs and lower back. Ideally, your thighs should be parallel to the floor. If your chair lacks adjustability, a footrest might help.

- **Back Support:** Look for a chair that provides **lumbar support**—a cushion that fits into the lower curve of your back. This helps reduce strain on the spine. If your chair doesn't offer adequate support, consider using a small pillow or lumbar roll to help maintain the natural curve of your back.

- **Seat Depth:** The depth of the seat should allow you to sit all the way back, so your back is fully supported. Make sure there's about 2-4 inches between the edge of the seat and the back of your knees.

- **Armrests:** The armrests should be positioned so that your shoulders remain relaxed and your elbows form a 90-degree angle. If the armrests are too high or too low, it can cause strain on the shoulders and neck.

3. Desk And Monitor Setup

Once you've ensured that your chair is properly adjusted, the next step is to focus on your desk and monitor setup. If the desk is too high or too low, or if the monitor is positioned improperly, it can strain your neck, shoulders, and eyes. Here are the key elements to get right:

- **Desk Height:** Your desk should allow your forearms to be parallel to the ground when typing, and your hands should float comfortably above the keyboard. Your elbows should remain at a 90-degree angle to avoid straining your wrists.

- **Monitor Position:** The top of the monitor should be at or slightly below eye level. Looking up or down at the screen for extended periods can lead to neck strain. The screen should also be about 20 to 30 inches away from your eyes. The angle of the screen should tilt slightly upward to reduce glare and prevent awkward head movements.

- **Keyboard And Mouse Placement:** Place your keyboard directly in front of you, ensuring your arms are at a comfortable angle. The mouse should be within easy reach and at the same height as the keyboard to avoid unnecessary shoulder and wrist strain.

4. Lighting And Screen Settings

Poor lighting and improper screen settings can lead to eye fatigue, headaches, and general discomfort. As a pain physician, I see many patients who report eye strain and tension headaches as a result of spending hours in front of bright screens in dimly lit rooms. Here's how to reduce those issues:

- **Lighting:** Ensure your workspace is well-lit, ideally with natural light. Position your desk so that sunlight doesn't create glare on your screen. If your workspace lacks natural light, use **task lighting** to reduce eye strain, and position it so it doesn't shine directly onto the screen.

- **Screen Brightness:** Adjust the brightness of your monitor to match the lighting conditions in the room. If the screen is too bright, it can strain your eyes; if it's too dim, it can cause you to lean forward, putting strain on your neck and back. Use the **blue light filter** to reduce eye fatigue, especially during long sessions at the computer.

- **Breaks And Eye Care:** Every 20-30 minutes, take a short break to look at something 20 feet away for 20 seconds. This can help reduce eye strain and prevent headaches, a simple but highly effective technique to avoid discomfort.

5. Posture And Movement

Even with an ergonomically optimized workspace, sitting for extended periods can still lead to discomfort. It's important to change positions frequently, stand up, and stretch. These movements reduce stiffness and keep the body in motion, which is crucial for pain prevention.

- **Sit Upright:** Keep your back straight, shoulders relaxed, and elbows close to your body. Avoid slouching or leaning forward, as this can cause strain in the back and neck. Consider using a lumbar roll or cushion to encourage good posture.

- **Change Positions Frequently:** Sitting for hours can lead to stiffness and discomfort. Aim to stand or move around every 30 to 60 minutes. Stretching, walking around, or even using a **standing desk** can help alleviate tension in your muscles and joints.

- **Stretching:** Take time to stretch your wrists, shoulders, and back to reduce muscle stiffness. Simple stretches throughout the day can go a long way in preventing pain and improving circulation.

6. Creating An Ergonomic Home Workspace

With the rise of remote work, many of us now spend hours working from home. However, home setups are often less ergonomic than office environments. Here's how to set up a more ergonomic workspace at home:

- Choose a **desk or table** that supports your posture and allows you to keep your body in alignment.

- If you don't have an ergonomic chair, use cushions or pillows to improve support.

- Consider using a **laptop stand** and external mouse and keyboard to adjust your screen and typing posture.

Conclusion

Incorporating **ergonomics** into your workspace can significantly reduce pain and discomfort, leading to improved well-being and productivity. Whether at the office or working from home, small changes—such as adjusting your chair height, optimizing your monitor setup, and taking regular breaks—can make a world of difference. A pain-free workspace not only helps you work more efficiently, but it also keeps your body healthy in the long run.

As a pain physician, my advice is to be mindful of your posture, listen to your body, and make the necessary adjustments to your workspace. By doing so, you'll be able to create a more comfortable and pain-free working environment.

10.3 The Role of Physical Activity

From the moment we begin our journey in the womb, our bodies are in motion. The foetus, even in the early stages of development, is actively moving and stretching within the protective confines of the womb. This constant motion is an essential part of our development, helping to build the foundation of our muscles, joints, and bones. As we transition into the world and grow, physical activity remains a crucial element of our well-being.

Throughout life, movement becomes the cornerstone of health. The role of physical activity in managing pain and improving overall health cannot be overstated. As a pain management specialist, I frequently emphasize to my patients that movement is not just about exercise—it is a vital component of maintaining and improving the function of the body, especially when dealing with chronic pain.

Why Physical Activity Matters in Pain Management

Physical activity plays a significant role in both preventing and managing pain. It is important to understand that, when done correctly, physical activity can act as a natural painkiller. Exercise helps by:

1. **Releasing Endorphins:** Physical activity triggers the release of endorphins, the body's natural pain-relieving chemicals. Endorphins work similarly to pain medications by reducing pain perception and improving mood.

2. **Reducing Inflammation:** Regular movement helps reduce the inflammation that can contribute to pain, particularly in conditions like arthritis. Exercise helps maintain joint flexibility and prevents the stiffness that worsens pain over time.

3. **Improving Circulation:** Physical activity enhances blood flow, which in turn delivers nutrients to tissues and removes waste products. This improves healing and reduces the pain associated with poor circulation, especially in injured muscles and joints.

4. **Strengthening Muscles and Joints:** Engaging in physical activity builds muscle strength, which provides better support to joints and reduces the risk of injury. Strong muscles help to stabilize joints and prevent the repetitive strain that leads to chronic pain, such as back pain or knee pain.

5. **Reducing Muscle Tension:** Many individuals who suffer from chronic pain also have muscle tightness and tension. Physical activity, particularly stretching and yoga, can help reduce this muscle tension, leading to better mobility and less discomfort.

Types Of Physical Activity for Pain Relief

The key to using physical activity as a tool for pain relief is to choose the right kind of movement and to do it in the right way. Here are some of the most effective types of physical activity for managing pain:

- **Low-Impact Exercise:** Activities like swimming, cycling, or walking are gentle on the joints but still offer significant benefits for pain relief. These exercises help to keep the body moving without placing undue stress on the joints or muscles, making them ideal for individuals with arthritis, fibromyalgia, or joint pain.

- **Strength Training:** Building strength is vital in pain management. Strengthening the muscles around painful joints provides stability, reducing the strain on the joints and improving overall function. Resistance training can also boost bone density, which is particularly beneficial for those with osteoarthritis or osteoporosis.

- **Stretching And Flexibility Exercises:** Stretching can improve the flexibility of muscles and joints, which is crucial for managing pain. Yoga and Pilates are excellent examples of activities that combine stretching with strength-building, promoting better posture, and reducing tension in the body.

- **Balance And Coordination Training:** Improving balance and coordination can prevent falls and injuries, which are common concerns for people experiencing chronic pain. Exercises that improve balance, such as tai chi, can also help with pain management, particularly for individuals with conditions like knee pain or back pain.

- **Mind-Body Exercises:** Practices like **yoga, tai chi**, and **qigong** are perfect examples of mind-body exercises that integrate gentle movement with relaxation techniques. These exercises are particularly beneficial for people dealing with chronic pain because they promote flexibility, reduce muscle tension, and help manage stress—one of the key contributors to pain.

The Psychological Benefits of Physical Activity

While the physical benefits of exercise are often the focus, it is essential to acknowledge the psychological advantages as well. Chronic pain is not only a physical challenge but also an emotional and mental one. The toll that constant pain can take on a person's mental well-being is profound. Anxiety, depression, and stress are common among those living with pain, and these psychological factors can, in turn, exacerbate the pain itself.

Physical activity is one of the most effective ways to combat the psychological effects of chronic pain. Exercise can:

- **Improve Mood:** As mentioned, the endorphins released during physical activity help elevate mood and reduce stress, anxiety, and depression. Regular exercise is associated with better mental health outcomes and increased overall happiness.

- **Boost Self-Confidence:** Physical activity can help patients regain their independence and confidence by improving physical function and reducing pain. The sense of accomplishment from being able to perform tasks that were previously difficult or impossible can be empowering.

- **Decrease Stress:** Stress is a major contributor to pain, as it can increase muscle tension and inflammation. Physical activity helps reduce stress and promotes relaxation, which is essential for both mental and physical well-being.

Overcoming Barriers to Physical Activity

For many people living with chronic pain, the idea of engaging in physical activity can seem daunting. Pain often leads to fear of worsening symptoms, and the thought of exercise might feel overwhelming. However, starting slowly and gradually increasing intensity can help alleviate these concerns. Here are some tips to help overcome barriers to exercise:

- **Start Small:** Begin with low-intensity activities, such as walking or gentle stretching. Gradually increase the duration and intensity as you build strength and tolerance. Consistency is key—small, regular movements are more effective than occasional intense exercise.

- **Listen To Your Body:** It's essential to pay attention to your body's signals. If something feels too intense, adjust the activity or take a break. It's okay to modify your routine to fit your current ability and comfort level.

- **Work With a Professional:** If you're unsure where to start, working with a physical therapist or pain specialist can help you develop a tailored exercise program that addresses your specific needs and limitations.

Conclusion

Physical activity is one of the most powerful tools available for managing pain and improving overall health. It's not just about fitness or weight loss; it's about maintaining a functional body and mind. As we move from the moment we are born, our bodies are designed to be in motion. By staying active, we maintain our muscles, joints, and overall health, preventing injury and alleviating chronic pain.

As a pain physician, I cannot stress enough the importance of physical activity. It doesn't matter if you're living with chronic pain or just trying to maintain your health—movement is the key. The best part is that it's never too late to start. So, get moving today, listen to your body, and make physical activity a part of your daily routine. Your body and mind will thank you for it.

10.4 Quality Sleep and Its Impact on Pain Relief

Sleep is not just a time for rest; it is a crucial period of healing and recovery. When we sleep, our bodies undergo essential processes that promote tissue repair, reduce inflammation, and regulate pain. Unfortunately, chronic pain often disrupts sleep, creating a vicious cycle that exacerbates both the pain and the inability to rest. As a pain management specialist, I see firsthand how the lack of quality sleep can worsen symptoms, making it harder for patients to manage their pain.

The Connection Between Sleep and Pain

The relationship between sleep and pain is complex, with each influencing the other. On one hand, poor sleep can increase the perception of pain, while on the other, it can interfere with the ability to fall and stay asleep. Here's why sleep is vital for managing pain:

1. **Healing And Tissue Repair:** During deep sleep, the body engages in repair and regeneration. Muscles and joints that have been overworked or injured need time to heal, and sleep is essential for this process. Growth hormone, which is released during sleep, plays a significant role in tissue repair, helping the body recover from pain or injury.

2. **Reduction In Inflammation:** Chronic pain conditions, such as arthritis or fibromyalgia, often involve inflammation. Sleep helps regulate the body's inflammatory response, lowering the levels of pro-inflammatory cytokines that can increase pain sensitivity. Quality sleep ensures that the body remains in a state of healing and recovery.

3. **Pain Sensitivity and Pain Perception:** Lack of sleep amplifies the brain's response to pain. When you don't get enough rest, your nervous system becomes more sensitive, which means that even minor pain signals can feel much more intense. Sleep deprivation leads to a heightened perception of pain, making even normal discomfort feel unbearable.

4. **Mood And Stress Regulation:** Chronic pain often leads to stress, anxiety, and depression. Unfortunately, these emotional factors can disrupt sleep, leading to a cycle of increased pain and worsening mental health. Quality sleep plays a vital role in regulating mood and reducing stress hormones such as cortisol, which can worsen pain perception.

Improving Sleep Quality for Pain Relief

For those who suffer from chronic pain, sleep may feel elusive. However, some steps can be taken to improve sleep quality and break the cycle of pain and insomnia:

1. **Create A Sleep-Friendly Environment:** Your sleep environment should be conducive to relaxation and comfort. This means a dark, quiet room with a comfortable mattress and pillow. Reducing environmental stressors, such as excessive noise or bright lights, can help signal to your body that it's time to wind down.

2. **Establish A Sleep Routine:** Try to go to bed and wake up at the same time every day, even on weekends. Consistency helps regulate the body's internal clock, improving the quality of sleep over time. Engaging in a pre-bedtime routine, such as reading a book or taking a warm bath, can signal to the body that it's time to sleep.

3. **Avoid Stimulants:** Caffeine, nicotine, and heavy meals close to bedtime can interfere with your ability to fall asleep. Avoid these stimulants, especially in the hours leading up to bedtime. Alcohol may make you feel sleepy initially but can disrupt sleep later in the night, leading to poor rest and more pain.

4. **Practice Relaxation Techniques:** Stress and anxiety can prevent restful sleep. Techniques such as deep breathing, progressive muscle relaxation, or mindfulness meditation can calm the nervous system and promote better sleep. Consider using guided meditation apps or listening to soothing music before bed to help you relax.

5. **Address Pain Before Bedtime:** If pain is preventing you from falling asleep, consider taking steps to manage it before bed. Apply heat or cold packs, practice gentle stretches, or take a warm bath to relax your muscles. Pain management treatments, such as physical therapy or medications, can help reduce discomfort, allowing for a more restful night.

6. **Exercise Regularly:** Regular physical activity helps regulate sleep patterns and reduces pain sensitivity. However, it is important to avoid intense workouts too close to bedtime, as this can have the opposite effect and interfere with sleep. Aim for moderate exercise earlier in the day to help improve both pain levels and sleep quality.

The Bottom Line on Sleep and Pain Relief

Quality sleep is an integral part of managing pain. Whether you're dealing with chronic conditions like arthritis or recovering from an injury, sleep provides the foundation for your body to heal and regenerate. By making sleep a priority and adopting strategies to improve sleep quality, you can break the cycle of pain and sleeplessness and feel better both physically and mentally.

10.5 Preventing Pain Through Daily Habits

Prevention is always better than cure, and this rings especially true when it comes to pain management. While it may not always be possible to avoid pain entirely, adopting healthy daily habits can significantly reduce the risk of pain and discomfort in the long term. As a pain physician, my focus is not only on treating existing pain but also on helping patients build a lifestyle that prevents future injuries and pain flare-ups.

The good news is that small changes in daily habits can have a profound impact on pain prevention. By integrating these simple practices into your routine, you can protect your joints, muscles, and bones, reduce your risk of developing chronic pain, and improve your overall well-being.

1. Maintaining Proper Posture

One of the most effective ways to prevent pain, especially in the back, neck, and joints, is to maintain good posture throughout the day. Poor posture, whether sitting, standing, or sleeping, places unnecessary strain on muscles and joints, leading to discomfort and pain.

- **At Your Desk:** Ensure that your chair supports the natural curve of your spine, and keep your feet flat on the ground. Your screen should be at eye level, and your arms should rest comfortably at a 90-degree angle. Avoid slouching or leaning forward, which can put stress on your back.

- **When Standing:** Distribute your weight evenly between both legs, with your shoulders aligned over your hips and your head held upright. Avoid locking your knees or leaning to one side.

- **When Sleeping:** Use a supportive pillow and mattress that help maintain the natural curve of your spine. Sleeping on your side with a pillow between your knees can help prevent lower back pain.

2. Stay Active

As discussed earlier, regular physical activity is essential for preventing pain. Movement keeps your muscles, joints, and bones strong and flexible. Incorporating daily movement into your routine—whether it's walking, stretching, or strength training—helps prevent stiffness, improve circulation, and reduce the risk of injury.

- **Stretching:** Incorporating a few minutes of stretching into your daily routine helps maintain flexibility and range of motion. Focus on areas prone to tightness, such as your neck, shoulders, back, and hips.

- **Strengthening Exercises:** Building muscle strength, especially in the core, back, and legs, provides better support for your spine and joints, reducing the risk of injuries and pain.

3. Pay Attention to Ergonomics

Whether you're working at a desk, lifting objects, or even driving, proper ergonomics can prevent strain and injury. Here are a few tips for preventing pain through better ergonomics:

- **At Work:** Set up your workspace to support proper posture and movement. Adjust the height of your desk, chair, and computer screen so that your body is in a neutral position.

- **When Lifting:** Always use your legs, not your back, to lift heavy objects. Keep the load close to your body and avoid twisting your torso while lifting.

4. Stay Hydrated and Eat Well

Nutrition plays a key role in pain prevention. Eating a balanced diet rich in vitamins, minerals, and anti-inflammatory foods can reduce the risk of developing chronic pain conditions, such as arthritis. Omega-3 fatty acids, found in foods like salmon, flaxseeds, and walnuts, help reduce inflammation in the body.

Staying hydrated is also essential, as dehydration can lead to muscle cramps and joint stiffness, which may contribute to pain. Aim to drink plenty of water throughout the day to keep your muscles and joints well-lubricated.

5. Get Regular Check-Ups

Preventive healthcare is critical for avoiding pain. Regular check-ups with your doctor, physical therapist, or chiropractor can help identify potential issues before they become serious problems. Early intervention is key to preventing the progression of musculoskeletal conditions or injuries.

6. Manage Stress

Stress is a major contributor to physical tension, which can lead to muscle pain and headaches. Incorporating stress-reducing practices such as deep breathing, meditation, or mindfulness into your daily routine can help prevent pain caused by tension and anxiety.

Conclusion

Making Prevention Part of Your Lifestyle

Preventing pain is all about making small, sustainable changes to your daily habits. By maintaining good posture, staying active, and focusing on ergonomics, nutrition, and stress management, you can significantly reduce your risk of developing pain and improve your overall quality of life. Just like you brush your teeth daily to prevent cavities, adopting these habits can help you maintain a pain-free and healthy body for years to come.

Part 5
Behind The Scenes in Medicine

Chapter 11
The Art of Diagnosis

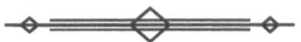

In the medical field, diagnosis is an art as much as it is science. As a doctor, I often tell my patients that the first step in understanding their condition is to listen. A thorough, empathetic listening session is invaluable—which not only builds trust but often holds the key to unlocking the cause of their symptoms. A clinical examination and tests are necessary, but they come after truly understanding the patient's story.

11.1 Listening to The Patient's Story

In my practice, I have learned time and again that the patient's narrative is just as important as the medical tests and imaging. The first consultation isn't just about running through a list of symptoms. It is about engaging with the patient, making them feel heard, and collecting the nuances of their experience that could provide clues to their diagnosis.

The Power of Listening

Listening to a patient isn't just about hearing the words they say, but also understanding the emotions behind those words. The story they tell gives insight into their journey with pain or illness and helps me form a more complete picture of their health.

When I sit down with a patient, I encourage them to share their symptoms in their own words—how the pain started, its intensity, what makes it better or worse, and how it impacts their daily life. This initial conversation is the foundation of the diagnostic process. Here's why listening is so essential in diagnosing accurately:

1. **Gaining Context**: A patient's symptoms alone may not always be enough to pinpoint a diagnosis. By asking open-ended questions and listening to the patient's story, I gain context that could reveal hidden factors, like lifestyle, environmental influences, or emotional triggers, which may be influencing their condition.

2. **Understanding The Journey**: Often, patients have seen multiple healthcare providers before they come to me. Their journey involves experiences with various tests, treatments, and outcomes. Listening carefully allows me to better understand what has been tried, what worked, and what didn't. This history is crucial in narrowing down potential causes and preventing unnecessary duplication of tests.

3. **Building Trust**: Empathy plays a key role in making the patient feel understood. Trust between the doctor and patient allows for more honest communication. When patients feel they are being heard and valued, they are more likely to share important details that could be crucial for

diagnosis. They may mention factors they didn't think were relevant or they may be more open to discussing sensitive issues, like emotional stress or lifestyle factors.

4. **Empathetic Approach**: Listening with empathy allows for the validation of a patient's pain or discomfort. Pain is a subjective experience, and no two individuals experience it in the same manner. Understanding a patient's emotional and psychological state can also inform the diagnosis—sometimes emotional distress manifests as physical pain or chronic stress could be contributing to the physical ailments.

5. **Creating A Collaborative Environment**: The diagnostic process is not just about the doctor taking decision based on tests and medical knowledge; it's about collaborating with the patient. Listening to their experiences and concerns helps me work together with them to explore different possibilities and find the most suitable course of action. It fosters a partnership where the patient feels empowered and actively involved in their treatment plan.

Practical Approaches to Listening Effectively

1. **Active Listening:** When I'm with a patient, I practice active listening. This means that I focus completely on the patient's words, avoiding interruptions, and responding thoughtfully. I maintain eye contact, nod in agreement, and ask

clarifying questions if necessary to show that I am engaged.

2. **Creating A Comfortable Environment:** A sterile, clinical setting can sometimes make patients feel nervous or guarded. I aim to create a welcoming, relaxed environment where patients feel comfortable sharing their concerns openly. This includes offering reassurance when needed, using a calm tone of voice, and making sure they know they have my full attention.

3. **Non-Verbal Cues:** Pay attention to body language—both the patient's and your own. A patient's posture, facial expressions, and tone of voice often provide valuable information beyond words. Likewise, my body language—such as sitting at eye level with the patient, avoiding distractions, and maintaining a supportive posture—can make a big difference in fostering trust and open communication.

4. **Open-Ended Questions:** Instead of asking yes-or-no questions, I prefer to ask open-ended questions such as "Can you describe how the pain feels?" or "How does this impact your daily routine?" This encourages the patient to share more detailed and specific information.

5. **Allowing Silence:** Sometimes, patients may need a moment to gather their thoughts or process their emotions. I try not to rush them or fill every pause with words. Allowing moments of silence can

give the patient the space they need to share additional important details.

How Listening Leads to Accurate Diagnosis

A clear diagnosis stems from understanding the full context of a patient's condition. Once I have listened to their story, I can complement it with diagnostic tests, physical exams, and further questioning to form a comprehensive picture. For example, a patient might describe back pain that has been present for months. Upon listening, I discovered that the pain worsens with prolonged sitting at work and is accompanied by numbness in their legs. With this information, I might consider issues like herniated discs or sciatica and proceed to confirm this diagnosis through imaging and tests.

In some cases, patients' stories might lead to a more holistic diagnosis. For instance, someone experiencing chronic pain in multiple joints might not just have osteoarthritis but could also be suffering from an autoimmune condition. In this case, their narrative allows me to think beyond the obvious and explore other possibilities.

Conclusion

Diagnosis Is a Journey, Not Just A Label

As a doctor, I always remind myself that every patient is unique. Their pain, experiences, and symptoms cannot always be understood from a textbook or a set of lab results alone. Listening to their story is an essential part of uncovering the truth behind their condition. It's through this dialogue that I can guide them on the road to healing, offering them the best possible chance at recovery.

By treating the patient as a partner in the diagnostic process, we not only work toward a correct diagnosis but also build the trust and empathy needed for a successful treatment plan. After all, medicine is not just about fixing problems—it's about understanding people, their struggles, and their lives.

11.2 Identifying Patterns and Rare Conditions

In medicine, one of the most critical skills I've developed over the years is recognizing patterns in patient symptoms. Patterns can offer crucial indicators for diagnosis, aiding in the identification of not only common conditions but also rare and complex ones that could otherwise go unnoticed.

As a pain specialist, this is especially important because pain can be a symptom of so many different disorders, some of which are much more elusive.

The Importance of Recognizing Patterns

When a patient presents with a set of symptoms, the first thing I do is look for patterns. Every patient's story is unique, and by carefully listening and observing their symptoms, I can detect recurrent trends that point to a particular diagnosis. Patterns can emerge from the timing, intensity, location, and nature of the pain itself. The way pain behaves can sometimes tell me more than any test result.

For instance, in musculoskeletal pain, patients might describe pain that intensifies at certain times of day or after specific activities. If a patient with chronic knee pain describes pain that worsens after climbing stairs but improves after rest, this could point to osteoarthritis. If the pain is present at all times and doesn't improve with rest, we might start thinking about other causes like inflammatory arthritis.

Recognizing these patterns early in the diagnostic process can be a game-changer. It guides my decision-making and helps me decide which tests to order or which specialists to consult.

Identifying Rare Conditions

While most pain physicians deal with common ailments like osteoarthritis, back pain, or musculoskeletal strains, my training and experience have made me aware of the importance of recognizing rare conditions. Rare diseases often don't present with clear, telltale signs, which means they can easily be misdiagnosed or dismissed.

One example from my practice that comes to mind is **Ehlers-Danlos syndrome** (EDS), a connective tissue disorder that causes joints to become hypermobile, leading to chronic pain and frequent dislocations. It's not something every doctor thinks about when someone walks in complaining of joint pain, but the key to identifying it lies in recognizing certain patterns of hypermobility, bruising, and skin elasticity—patterns that aren't common in typical joint pain cases.

Similarly, conditions like **Complex Regional Pain Syndrome** (CRPS) or **fibromyalgia** can be difficult to diagnose at first because they don't show up clearly in lab tests or imaging. CRPS, for example, is often triggered by an injury but results in prolonged, severe pain that spreads beyond the injury site. Fibromyalgia is characterized by widespread pain, fatigue, and tender points throughout the body but lacks objective findings that can easily confirm the diagnosis. The key to identifying these conditions often lies in recognizing the pattern of symptoms and ruling out other possibilities.

When a patient presents with symptoms that don't fit neatly into any known category, it requires a careful and thoughtful approach. I've had patients who initially seemed to be dealing with simple back pain, but after a thorough history and physical exam, I recognized a rare case of **ankylosing spondylitis** (AS), a type of arthritis that affects the spine and can cause severe pain and stiffness. Recognizing the early signs allows better treatment, improving the patient's quality of life.

The Role Of A Comprehensive History And Physical Exam

To identify rare conditions, a comprehensive history and physical exam are crucial. Sometimes, rare conditions might have subtle signs that are only noticeable if you know what to look for. I rely heavily on asking detailed questions about the patient's family history, lifestyle, and any previous conditions they may have experienced. For example, if a patient reports a history of frequent joint dislocations or if they mention that their skin is unusually stretchy or fragile, I might suspect a connective tissue disorder like EDS, prompting further tests.

It's also important to use a systematic approach when examining patients. I follow a structured process that looks at all the potential causes of pain, including neurological, musculoskeletal, and inflammatory factors. This broad approach ensures that I don't miss a rare condition just because it doesn't fit the typical mould.

Collaborating With Specialists

When a rare condition is suspected, I often collaborate with other specialists to confirm the diagnosis. This might include a rheumatologist for autoimmune or inflammatory disorders, a neurologist for conditions like multiple sclerosis or neuropathy, or a geneticist for inherited diseases. In some cases, advanced imaging, genetic testing, or referral to tertiary care centres may be necessary.

One of the challenges in diagnosing rare conditions is that many of them have overlapping symptoms with more common disorders. For example, **multiple sclerosis** can sometimes present with pain, muscle weakness, and fatigue, symptoms that are similar to those seen in chronic fatigue syndrome or fibromyalgia. In these cases, careful pattern recognition, along with specialized tests like MRI scans, can help us make the correct diagnosis.

Patterns In Chronic Pain Syndromes

Another area where recognizing patterns is crucial is in managing chronic pain syndromes. Chronic pain often doesn't have an obvious cause, and there are many factors that can contribute to its persistence, including emotional stress, genetics, and lifestyle factors.

I often see patients who have been suffering from chronic pain for months or even years without any clear diagnosis. Their symptoms may not point to a single disease but rather a complex interaction of physical, psychological, and environmental factors. For example, **chronic low back pain** might be due to a variety of factors, such as degenerative disc disease, muscle strain, or even emotional stress. In these cases, identifying the pattern of symptoms—when they worsen, how they respond to treatment, and any other contributing factors—helps me craft a treatment plan that addresses all aspects of the condition.

In these situations, patient collaboration is key. By discussing their symptoms in detail and recognizing patterns in their pain, we can develop a plan that not only treats the physical aspects of it but also addresses lifestyle factors like stress, sleep, and exercise.

Conclusion

The Art of Diagnosing Rare Conditions

Identifying rare conditions requires a blend of knowledge, experience, and intuition. It's not enough to just look at the patient's symptoms in isolation—what matters is the bigger picture. By carefully listening to the patient, observing patterns in their symptoms, and using a systematic approach to diagnosis, I can uncover conditions that might not be immediately obvious.

In medicine, especially in pain management, it's crucial to remember that every patient is unique. They may present with a rare condition, or they may have a common condition that behaves uncommonly. By developing a keen eye for patterns, continuously expanding my knowledge, and working closely with other specialists, I can ensure that every patient receives the best possible care, no matter how rare or complex their condition may be.

Chapter 12
The Business of Healthcare

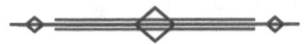

12.1 Challenges of Running A Pain Clinic

Running a pain clinic is not just about providing treatment; it's about striking a delicate balance between offering top-notch care, managing business operations, and navigating the complex healthcare ecosystem. As the head of the Praanaa pain clinic, I've come to realize that the challenges of running a clinic often extend far beyond the examination room.

1. **Delivering Quality Care Amid Financial Constraints:** One of the biggest hurdles is ensuring that every patient receives the best care possible while operating within financial limits. Healthcare is expensive—medical equipment, diagnostic tools, medications, and staff salaries all that contributes to the cost of running a clinic. For a pain clinic, where patients often require ongoing treatments like physical therapy, injections, or advanced interventions, managing these costs without compromising quality is a constant challenge

2. Insurance reimbursements often don't align with the actual costs of care. For instance, some procedures may be reimbursed at rates that barely cover the expenses involved, leaving the clinic to absorb the loss. This makes it essential to streamline operations and optimize resources while maintaining the highest standards of care.

3. **Navigating Patient Expectations and Satisfaction:** Patients who visit pain clinics often come with high expectations—they are seeking relief from chronic pain that has persisted despite previous treatments. Meeting these expectations while being transparent about what is realistically achievable requires clear communication and empathy.

4. For example, some patients expect immediate relief after a single treatment. As a practitioner, it's my responsibility to explain that chronic pain often requires a multi-faceted and long-term approach. Balancing patient satisfaction while setting realistic goals is both a clinical and a business challenge.

5. **Keeping Up with Medical Advancements:** Pain management is a rapidly evolving field, with new treatments, technologies, and research emerging every year. Staying up-to-date with these advancements is essential to offering cutting-edge care to patients. However, adopting new technologies or treatments often comes with

significant costs, both in terms of purchasing equipment and training staff.

6. For instance, implementing radiofrequency ablation or regenerative therapies like platelet-rich plasma (PRP) requires not only investment in technology but also specialized training. Deciding when and how to integrate these advancements into the clinic's offerings is a strategic challenge that requires careful planning.

7. **Regulatory And Compliance Challenges:** Healthcare is one of the most heavily regulated industries. Pain clinics, in particular, face stringent regulations to prevent the misuse of medications like opioids. While these regulations are essential for patient safety, they also add layers of administrative work and legal scrutiny.

8. For example, prescribing controlled substances for chronic pain requires meticulous documentation and compliance with government guidelines. Any oversight, even unintentional, can result in audits, penalties, or even legal action. Managing these compliance requirements while ensuring smooth day-to-day operations is a constant juggling act.

9. **Building And Retaining a Competent Team:** A pain clinic's success depends heavily on its team—doctors, nurses, physical therapists, administrative staff, and more. Recruiting skilled professionals who share the clinic's vision and

retaining them in a competitive healthcare environment is no small feat.

10. Burnout is a significant issue in pain management, not just for doctors but for the entire team. Dealing with patients in chronic pain can be emotionally taxing, and it's important to foster a supportive and collaborative work environment. Regular training, recognition, and opportunities for professional growth are essential to keep the team motivated and engaged.

11. **Patient Accessibility and Outreach:** Another challenge is making the clinic accessible to as many patients as possible, especially in underserved areas where specialized pain management services are scarce. Marketing the clinic's services without falling into the trap of overpromising is a delicate task.

12. For example, some clinics advertise miraculous results, which can mislead patients and erode trust in the medical profession. I firmly believe that marketing should be ethical, focusing on what we can realistically deliver.

13. **Balancing Business Goals with Patient Care:** Perhaps the most difficult challenge of all is striking a balance between the financial goals of running a clinic and the core mission of helping patients. In today's healthcare environment, there's often pressure to increase patient volume or promote high-revenue procedures. However,

this should never come at the expense of patient-centred care.

14. In my clinic, we prioritize a personalized approach, tailoring treatments to each patient's unique needs rather than pushing one-size-fits-all solutions. While this may not always be the most profitable approach in the short term, it builds trust and ensures long-term success.

Conclusion

A Delicate Balancing Act of running a pain clinic is as much about strategy and resilience as it is about medicine. It requires a deep commitment to patient care, a willingness to adapt to challenges, and a strong sense of purpose. For me, the ultimate reward lies in seeing patients regain their quality of life—a goal that makes every challenge worth overcoming.

12.2 The Economics of Non-Surgical Treatments

Non-surgical treatments for pain management have gained significant traction as patients increasingly seek effective alternatives to invasive procedures. While these approaches often present numerous advantages, it's essential to clarify that they don't entirely replace the need for surgeries. Instead, they provide an opportunity to delay or avoid surgical interventions in certain cases where non-invasive methods are effective.

Let's explore how non-surgical treatments compare economically and where they fit within the broader scope of pain management.

1. Lower Immediate Costs Compared to Surgery

Surgical procedures are expensive, often due to the comprehensive nature of their delivery.

- **Operating** room charges, surgical team fees, and anaesthesia.
- Hospital stays for recovery and associated post-operative care.

For example, a knee replacement surgery could cost several lakhs, factoring in pre-surgical diagnostics and post-surgical rehabilitation. Non-surgical options—like nerve blocks, physical therapy, or PRP (platelet-rich plasma) therapy—are outpatient treatments, often performed at a fraction of the cost. Even with multiple sessions, these options remain more affordable in the short term.

2. Avoiding Unnecessary Surgical Interventions

It's important to acknowledge that not every case of chronic pain or joint dysfunction requires surgery. For conditions like mild to moderate osteoarthritis, soft tissue injuries, or nerve pain, evidence-backed non-surgical treatments can offer significant relief, potentially saving patients from unnecessary operations.

However, this doesn't mean surgeries are unnecessary in all situations. For advanced conditions like severe joint degeneration, fractures, or certain spinal pathologies, surgery remains the best and often the only solution. Non-surgical approaches serve as complementary options, providing relief and improving quality of life until surgery becomes unavoidable or as part of post-surgical rehabilitation.

3. Reduced Indirect Costs

Surgical procedures often incur hidden costs beyond the immediate financial burden, such as:

- **Time off work** due to prolonged recovery periods.
- **Rehabilitation programs** to regain mobility and strength.
- Potential **complications or revision surgeries**, adding to overall expenses.

Non-surgical treatments, in contrast, allow patients to recover faster and return to their daily lives sooner. This minimizes indirect costs like lost income or caregiver support, making them a cost-effective alternative in many cases.

4. Insurance And Affordability

While surgeries are often covered by insurance, they may still leave patients with high out-of-pocket expenses due to co-pays, deductibles, or coverage limits. Non-surgical treatments like physiotherapy, regenerative therapies, or ultrasound-guided injections are increasingly being recognized by insurance providers, making them more accessible to patients.

Patients should consult their insurance policies to understand the extent of coverage for non-surgical interventions, as this can further enhance their affordability.

5. Long-Term Financial Benefits

One of the biggest arguments against non-surgical treatments is the perception that they require repeated sessions, which might add up over time. However, the reality is more nuanced.

- By delaying or avoiding surgery, patients can save significant costs associated with hospitalization, post-surgical care, and potential complications.
- For example, regular physiotherapy, combined with lifestyle adjustments, may extend the lifespan of a deteriorating joint, postponing knee replacement surgery for years.

When viewed from a long-term perspective, non-surgical treatments often emerge as a more financially sustainable option.

6. Educating Patients About the Balance

A common challenge lies in patient perception. Many patients believe that surgery is a definitive, one-time solution, while non-surgical treatments might seem less impactful. This can lead to premature surgical decisions when non-invasive methods could have achieved similar outcomes.

It's crucial to educate patients that non-surgical options don't aim to replace surgeries entirely but to optimize treatment strategies. For some, these treatments can effectively delay the need for surgery, while for others, they act as complementary therapies that enhance surgical outcomes or manage post-surgical pain.

7. The Bigger Picture: A Balanced Approach

Surgeries are not the enemy of non-surgical treatments, nor should they be seen as opposing options. Instead, they are tools in a continuum of care. For instance:

- Non-surgical interventions can address early-stage conditions, providing relief and delaying progression.
- When surgery is inevitable, these treatments can enhance pre-operative readiness and improve post-surgical recovery.

By adopting a balanced, patient-centric approach, we can ensure that the right treatment is delivered at the right time, avoiding unnecessary procedures while achieving optimal outcomes.

Conclusion

Cost-Effective Without Compromise

Non-surgical treatments offer a valuable, cost-effective pathway for many patients who are seeking pain relief. They provide substantial savings, faster recovery, and reduced risks in suitable cases. However, this doesn't diminish the importance of surgeries where they are genuinely required.

As a pain physician, my priority is to assess each patient's condition holistically. By starting with non-invasive, evidence-backed treatments and progressing toward surgical options only, when necessary, we can provide care that is both financially and medically sound. Together, non-surgical and surgical options form a comprehensive toolkit for pain management, tailored to the unique needs of each patient.

12.3 The Impact of Corporate Hospitals On Specialists

The rise of corporate hospitals has significantly reshaped the medical landscape, offering state-of-the-art infrastructure, streamlined operations, and multidisciplinary teams under one roof. However, their growing dominance has brought both opportunities and challenges for medical specialists, including pain physicians.

As someone who has worked closely with corporate setups, I've witnessed firsthand how these dynamic impact the practice of medicine, patient care, and professional autonomy. Let's explore these aspects in greater detail.

1. The Promise of Corporate Hospitals

Corporate hospitals have transformed healthcare by emphasizing innovation and accessibility. For specialists, they offer:

- **Advanced Technology:** Access to cutting-edge diagnostic tools, minimally invasive surgical equipment, and regenerative treatment options.
- **Multidisciplinary Collaboration:** Specialists can consult with peers from other fields, enabling holistic patient care.

- **Patient Volume and Diversity:** With larger footprints and marketing budgets, corporate hospitals attract diverse cases, providing specialists with exposure to a wide range of conditions.

- **Professional Growth:** Opportunities for career advancement, training, and research collaborations are more readily available.

These factors make corporate hospitals appealing to both new and experienced specialists.

2. The Trade-Off: Autonomy Vs. Compliance

While corporate hospitals provide an enabling environment, they also come with their own set of restrictions:

- **Pressure to Meet Revenue Targets:** Specialists often face subtle (or overt) pressure to generate revenue through consultations, tests, or procedures. For pain physicians, this might mean recommending interventions like injections or regenerative therapies more frequently than necessary, which can conflict with ethical decision-making.

- **Protocol Over Personalization:** Standardized treatment pathways in corporate hospitals aim to ensure uniformity and efficiency, but they may leave little room for individualized care. Specialists might feel constrained by rigid guidelines that don't account for unique patient needs.

- **Time Constraints:** Specialists are expected to manage high patient volumes, often limiting the time they can spend on detailed consultations or follow-ups.

- **Referral Bias:** Internal policies may encourage referrals within the hospital's ecosystem, even if external specialists or smaller clinics might offer better solutions for the patient's condition.

3. Patient Perception: Trust Vs. Commercialization

Corporate hospitals often market themselves as premium care providers, which can influence how patients perceive their treatment.

- **Increased Expectations:** Patients assume that higher fees equate to better outcomes. This puts specialists under pressure to deliver immediate results, even in complex or chronic conditions like pain management, which require time and patient adherence.

- **Scepticism Toward Ethics:** Some patients perceive corporate hospitals as profit-driven, leading to mistrust in treatment recommendations. Specialists often find themselves justifying every decision to overcome this scepticism.

4. Competition Among Specialists

Corporate hospitals typically have large teams of specialists in the same field. While this fosters collaboration, it can also create internal competition.

- **Recognition Vs. Performance:** Specialists may feel overshadowed if their achievements are not adequately highlighted, or if internal hierarchies limit growth opportunities.

- **Unequal Case Distribution:** Senior specialists often receive priority in case referrals, while newer doctors might struggle to establish themselves.

5. The Influence on Pain Management Practices

For pain specialists, the corporate hospital model presents unique challenges:

- **Overemphasis On Procedures:** There can be an implicit push toward procedural interventions (like epidural injections or radiofrequency ablations) due to their profitability, even when conservative methods like physiotherapy or counselling could suffice.

- **Limited Scope for Holistic Care:** Pain management often requires a multidisciplinary approach, including lifestyle modifications and patient education. Corporate setups may prioritize interventions with immediate results, sidelining long-term strategies.

6. Navigating The Corporate Structure as A Specialist

Despite these challenges, specialists can thrive in corporate hospitals by adopting the right strategies:

- **Patient Advocacy:** Always prioritize patient welfare, even if it means navigating the hospital's policies tactfully. Ethical practice builds trust, both with patients and peers.

- **Focus On Evidence-Based Medicine:** Use clinical data to justify treatment plans. This not only aligns with ethical standards but also counters revenue-driven pressures.

- **Continuous Learning:** Leverage the resources and training programs offered by corporate hospitals to stay updated with the latest advancements.

- **Building A Personal Brand:** Develop a reputation for integrity and expertise within the hospital. This can help balance internal competition and establish authority.

7. The Bigger Picture: Collaboration or Conflict?

The relationship between specialists and corporate hospitals is complex. On one hand, these institutions provide the resources and patient base needed for specialists to excel. On the other hand, they challenge the autonomy and ethical framework of individual practitioners.

As a pain physician, I've learned that the key lies in maintaining a balance: leveraging the opportunities offered by corporate hospitals while staying true to the core principles of patient-centric care. It's not about rejecting the system but navigating it in a way that aligns with your professional values and ensures the best outcomes for your patients.

Conclusion

Corporate hospitals have undeniably reshaped modern healthcare, offering both benefits and challenges for specialists. By understanding and addressing these dynamics, specialists can not only survive but thrive, ensuring that the quality of care remains at the forefront in an increasingly commercialized environment.

12.4 Is Healthcare Becoming Too Commercial?

As a practising pain physician, I often encounter patients who feel that healthcare today is less about healing and more about profit. This growing perception raises an important question: Is healthcare becoming too commercialized?

To answer this, we must explore the delicate balance between business imperatives and the foundational purpose of medicine—to serve humanity.

1. The Rise of Healthcare As A Business

Healthcare has evolved into a massive global industry, with corporate hospitals, pharmaceutical companies, medical device manufacturers, and insurance firms all playing a role. While has this commercialization brought innovations and accessibility, it has also introduced business practices that sometimes overshadow patient care.

Key drivers of commercialization include:

- **Privatization Of Healthcare:** As public healthcare systems struggle to meet demand, private institutions have stepped in, often prioritizing revenue generation.

- **Profit Margins in Pharmaceuticals And Equipment:** Medications and advanced medical devices are priced with substantial profit margins, leading to skyrocketing costs for patients.

- **Insurance-Driven Decisions:** Insurance policies can dictate treatment options, sometimes limiting what physicians can offer based on cost considerations rather than patient needs.

2. The Patient's Perspective

Patients increasingly report feeling like "customers" rather than individuals seeking care. From hospital admissions to post-treatment billing, every step can feel transactional.

- **High Costs:** Routine consultations, diagnostic tests, and treatments can be prohibitively expensive, creating a perception that profit takes precedence over care.

- **Unnecessary Procedures:** There is concern that patients may be recommended tests, procedures, or treatments that are not medically necessary but generate revenue.

- **Confusion Over Costs:** Lack of transparency in billing further exacerbates distrust, with patients unsure of what they are paying for and why.

3. The Physician's Dilemma

Doctors, especially in corporate or private setups, often find themselves navigating a fine line between ethical care and meeting organizational goals. Some of the challenges include:

- **Pressure To Meet Targets:** Physicians may face subtle or overt expectations to increase patient volumes or perform more revenue-generating procedures.

- **Conflicted Decision-Making:** Balancing patient welfare with institutional demands can be emotionally and professionally taxing.

- **Time Constraints:** The need to see more patients in less time diminishes the quality of consultations and the physician-patient relationship.

4. The Consequences of Commercialization

The impact of excessive commercialization is felt across the healthcare spectrum:

- **Loss Of Trust:** Patients may distrust doctors and hospitals, questioning the necessity and cost of treatments.

- **Reduced Accessibility:** High costs can make quality healthcare unattainable for large sections of the population.
- **Ethical Erosion:** A system overly focused on profit risks compromising ethical standards and the core values of medicine.

5. Can Commercialization Be Balanced?

While commercialization brings undeniable challenges, it is also a reality that cannot be ignored. The key lies in finding a balance between financial sustainability and ethical care.

- **Transparency In Billing:** Clear communication about costs helps build trust and reduces patient anxiety.
- **Focus On Preventive Care:** Shifting from reactive treatments to preventive strategies can reduce costs while improving patient outcomes.
- **Promoting Evidence-Based Medicine:** Ensuring that all treatments and procedures are backed by science prevents unnecessary interventions.
- **Ethical Leadership:** Hospital administrators and policymakers must prioritize patient welfare alongside profitability.
- **Patient Education:** Empowering patients to ask questions and make informed decisions fosters collaboration and trust.

6. A Personal Perspective

As a pain physician, I have seen firsthand how commercialization affects patient care. For example, some patients hesitate to undergo essential diagnostic tests due to cost concerns, while others come with preconceived notions shaped by aggressive marketing campaigns for unnecessary treatments or supplements.

In my practice, I make a conscious effort to address these challenges:

- **Building Trust:** By explaining the rationale for every test or treatment and offering affordable alternatives wherever possible.
- **Encouraging Holistic Care:** Beyond medical interventions, I guide patients toward lifestyle changes that can enhance their overall health and reduce dependence on costly procedures.

While commercialization is an unavoidable reality, I believe that every physician has the power to prioritize patient welfare and lead by example.

Conclusion

Healthcare's commercial evolution is a double-edged sword. While it drives advancements and accessibility, unchecked profit motives can undermine its integrity. By fostering ethical practices, transparency, and patient-centred care, we can ensure that the medical field stays true to its mission of healing and compassion.

Part 6
Inspiration And Legacy

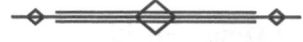

Chapter 13
Breaking The Pain Cycle

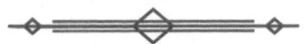

13.1 The Importance of Early Intervention

One of the most impactful lessons I've learned over the years is the importance of addressing pain early. The longer it persists, the harder it becomes to treat—not just physically, but mentally and emotionally too. Pain doesn't operate in isolation; it weaves into the fabric of your life, affecting your relationships, career, and overall well-being.

Why Do People Delay Seeking Help?

There are several reasons why patients delay getting treatment:

- **Misinformation:** A belief that pain will resolve on its own or is "part of ageing."

- **Denial:** People often downplay their discomfort, dismissing it as minor or manageable.

- **Fear Of Treatment:** Many assume that the only options involve invasive procedures like surgery.

- **Social Conditioning:** We live in a world where enduring pain is seen as a sign of strength, leading many to suffer silently.

However, this delay can have serious consequences. Chronic pain, if left untreated, can result in:

1. **Muscle Weakness or Joint Stiffness:** Making recovery more complex and time-consuming.

2. **Compensatory Pain:** Over time, your body develops secondary pain patterns in areas unaffected initially.

3. **Emotional Toll:** Anxiety, depression, and social isolation often accompany prolonged pain.

How Early Treatment Helps

Intervening early enables healthcare professionals to:

- Stop the pain before it worsens or spreads.
- Employ minimally invasive treatments, avoiding the need for costly and invasive surgery.
- Help patients maintain or regain mobility and independence.

For example, consider knee osteoarthritis—a common condition that starts as minor stiffness or discomfort. Addressing it early with weight management, specific exercises, and injectable treatments like viscosupplements can significantly delay the need for joint replacement surgery.

What You Can Do

If you experience pain, don't wait for it to escalate. Seek medical advice as soon as possible, and be open to exploring non-invasive options. Pain, when treated early, can become a manageable part of life rather than an all-consuming force.

13.2 Building A Support System for Chronic Pain Patients

Living with chronic pain can feel incredibly lonely. Many patients tell me that the most difficult part isn't the physical discomfort but the sense of isolation that comes with it. This is why having a strong support system is essential.

Support Starts at Home

Family members play an essential role in the journey of a pain patient. Their understanding, encouragement, and involvement can motivate them to keep going. However, this support needs to go beyond surface-level care.

- **Education:** Families must understand the nature of chronic pain, its unpredictability, and the fact that "pushing through" isn't always the answer.
- **Patience:** Pain isn't visible, making it easy to misunderstand. Listening without judgment is key.
- **Participation:** From attending medical appointments to helping with daily routines, small gestures of involvement can go a long way.

The Role of Healthcare Providers

Doctors, physiotherapists, and counsellors form another layer of support. A multidisciplinary approach ensures that patients receive holistic care, addressing not just physical pain but also mental and emotional struggles.

At **Praanaa**, we've taken steps to build communities for our patients. Through group counselling sessions, shared success stories, and online forums, we've created a safe space where individuals can connect and share experiences.

Empowering The Patient Community

When patients unite, magic happens. Communities of Chronic Pain sufferers provide a platform to:

- Share advice on managing daily challenges.
- Discuss new treatment options.
- Offer emotional support and encouragement.

These groups become a source of strength, reminding everyone involved that they're not alone in their journey.

13.3 Overcoming Stigma Around Pain and Treatment

Pain is often misunderstood—not just by those who experience it, but by society as a whole. Over the years, I've observed the many ways in which stigma stops people from seeking timely and appropriate care.

The Origins of Stigma

- **Cultural Perceptions:** Many cultures equate pain with weakness or view it as a test of endurance.

- **Judgment Of Pain Medications:** The misuse of painkillers has overshadowed their legitimate use, making many hesitant to consider them as an option.

- **Scepticism Around Non-Surgical Treatments:** People often view non-invasive treatments as "less effective," despite ample evidence to the contrary.

How To Combat These Misconceptions

Education and advocacy are critical in breaking down these barriers. As healthcare professionals, we must:

1. **Challenge Stereotypes:** Pain is not a moral failure but a medical condition deserving of treatment.

2. **Demystify Medications:** Helping patients understand the science behind pain medications can alleviate their fears.

3. **Promote Non-Surgical Solutions:** Sharing real-life success stories can inspire confidence in non-invasive options.

When stigma is removed, patients feel empowered to take control of their health without guilt or fear.

13.4 For All the Aspiring Doctors

As someone who has walked the path of medicine, I want to share a few heartfelt insights with those considering or beginning their journey in the medical profession. Being a doctor is one of the most rewarding careers, but it's also one of the most challenging. It requires not just knowledge and skill but an immense capacity for empathy, resilience, and perseverance.

The Calling

Medicine isn't just a career—it's a calling. It demands your time, energy, and dedication like few other professions. If you're drawn to this field because you genuinely want to help people, you're already on the right track. The road ahead will be tough, but your purpose will give you strength.

Lessons I've Learned

1. Listen More Than You Speak

Every patient has a story, and sometimes the key to their diagnosis lies not in their test results but in their words. Learn to listen deeply, not just to what they say, but to what they don't say.

2. Knowledge Is a Lifelong Pursuit

The field of medicine evolves rapidly. What you learn in medical school is just the foundation. Stay curious, stay updated, and never stop learning. Your willingness to grow will directly impact your ability to help patients.

3. Compassion Is Key

Patients don't just come to you for treatment—they come to you for hope. A kind word, a listening ear, or a moment of empathy can mean as much to them as a prescription or procedure.

4. Balance Is Crucial

Medicine can consume your life if you let it. Find ways to prioritize your mental and physical health. A burned-out doctor cannot provide the best care. Remember, you can only pour from a full cup.

5. Teamwork Makes the Dream Work

You will rarely work alone. Whether it's nurses, technicians, or specialists in other fields, respect and collaboration are essential. Medicine is a team effort, and every member of that team plays a critical role.

Challenges You'll Face

The Medical Profession Comes with Its Share of Challenges.

- Emotional Toll: You'll witness the suffering, loss, and sometimes the limits of what medicine can achieve.
- Long Hours: Medicine is a demanding field, and sacrifices are part of the job.
- The Pressure to Succeed: People will place immense trust in you, and that responsibility can make you feel overwhelming at times.

But remember, these challenges are also what makes the victories so much sweeter. The gratitude in a patient's eyes, the joy of a family reunited with their loved one, or the knowledge that your work has made a real difference—these moments will remind you why you chose this path.

To The Aspiring Specialists

If you're considering a specialization like pain management, know that it's one of the most fulfilling fields. Helping people find relief from chronic pain, restore their quality of life, and witness their transformation is an incredible privilege.

A Final Word of Encouragement

Medicine is not just about curing—it's about caring. It's about being a beacon of hope in someone's darkest hours. If you choose this path, do so with your whole heart. The road may be long and challenging, but the destination is worth every step.

The world needs more compassionate, dedicated doctors. If that's the kind of doctor you aspire to be, then I welcome you to this noble profession with open arms.

You have the power to change lives, one patient at a time. And in doing so, you'll find that the life you change the most is your own.

13.5 A Message of Hope

If you're living with pain, I want you to know this: there is hope. Pain might feel like an insurmountable force in your life, but it's not something you have to endure alone or indefinitely.

The Journey of Healing

Pain relief is not always instantaneous—it's a journey. Some days will be harder than others, but every step you take toward healing is a victory. Whether it's finding the right doctor, trying a new treatment, or simply sharing your experience with someone who understands, each effort brings you closer to relief.

Reflections On My Work

As a pain physician, I've had the privilege of witnessing countless transformations. Patients who thought they'd never walk again now dance at their children's weddings. Individuals who couldn't sleep through the night now wake up refreshed and ready to face the day. These stories fuel my passion and remind me of the power of perseverance.

My Promise to You

This book is more than just information—it's a commitment. A commitment to empower you with knowledge, debunk myths, and inspire you to take charge of your pain.

Pain doesn't have to control your life. With the right tools, mindset, and support, you can regain your independence and rediscover joy. Together, we can challenge misconceptions, explore innovative treatments, and embrace a future which would be free from pain.

Above all, remember this: you are not defined by your pain. You are defined by your resilience, your hope, and your willingness to seek a better tomorrow.

Let's build that tomorrow together.

www.ingramcontent.com/pod-product-compliance
Lightning Source LLC
LaVergne TN
LVHW091637070526
838199LV00044B/1099